# THE HIGH FIBER COOKBOOK

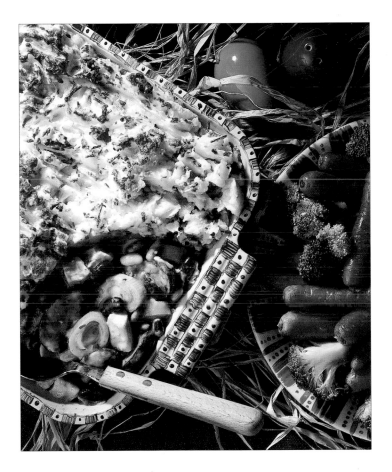

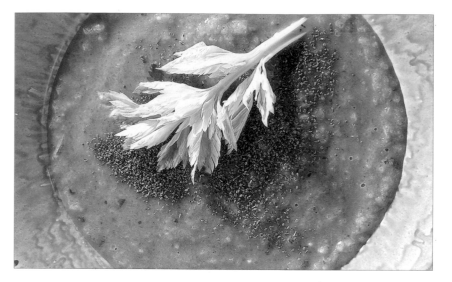

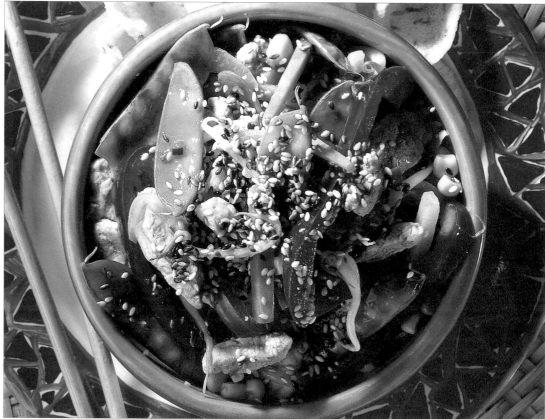

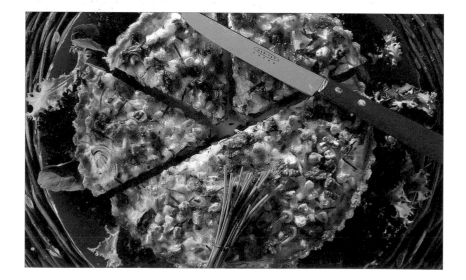

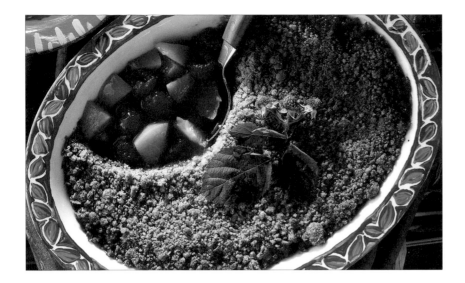

# THE HIGH FIBRE COOKBOOK

## OVER 50 DELICIOUS RECIPES FOR HEALTHY EATING

## ANNE SHEASBY

LORENZ BOOKS

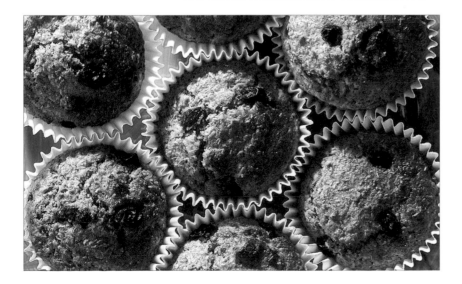

First published in 1999 by Lorenz Books

First published in 1998 by Lorenz Books
27 West 20th Street, New York, NY 10011

LORENZ BOOKS are available for bulk purchase for sales promotion and for
premium use. For details, write or call the sales director, Lorenz Books,
27 West 20th Street, New York, NY 10011; (800) 354-9657

Lorenz Books is an imprint of
Anness Publishing Inc.

ISBN 1 85967 883 1

*Publisher*: Joanna Lorenz
*Project Editor*: Zoe Antoniou
*Designer*: Ian Sandom
*Photographer*: David Jordan
*Additional Photographers*: Janine Hosegood (pp8, 10, 12 left) and Patrick McLeavey (pp12 right, 13)
*Illustrator*: Madeleine David
*Stylist*: Judy Williams
*Production Controller*: Joanna King

Previously published as *High Fiber Cookbook*

Printed and bound in Singapore

1 3 5 7 9 10 8 6 4 2

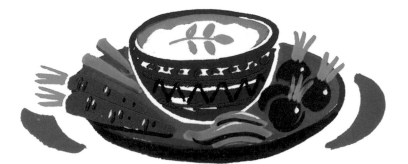

# CONTENTS

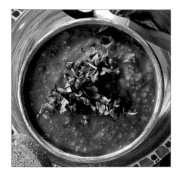

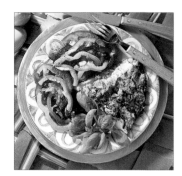

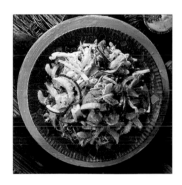

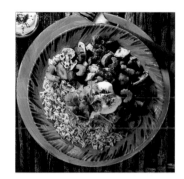

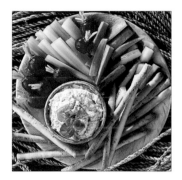

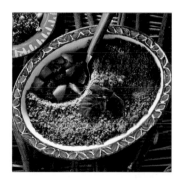

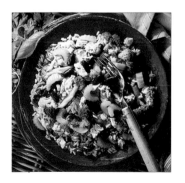

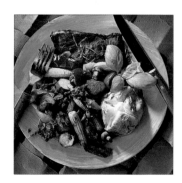

# INTRODUCTION

The importance of fiber in a healthy, balanced diet should not be underestimated. Once labeled "roughage" and thought of simply as a bulking agent, dietary fiber is increasingly seen as essential in preventing or at least alleviating a wide range of digestive disorders and is believed to help lower cholesterol levels and help prevent coronary heart disease.

Western man has gone soft—in dietary terms—swapping a diet that was high in fiber for one that relies heavily on processed low-fiber foods. It has been estimated that many of us consume no more than 11 grams of fiber a day, whereas the recommended daily intake is between 12 to 18 grams.

This book looks at all the advantages of increasing the amount of dietary fiber we consume and suggests a few simple changes that can be introduced over time to make a healthy, well-balanced diet even better. It includes a selection of tempting recipes, chosen first for flavor, second for fiber content and always for all-around appeal to every member of the family.

## THE IMPORTANCE OF FIBER

Changing to a diet that is higher in dietary fiber is not difficult, but it should be done gradually. Sudden and significant changes to your normal eating patterns may actually upset the digestive system.

Dietary fiber—or nonstarch polysaccharides (NSP), as it is more accurately described—is divided into two main types: soluble fiber and insoluble fiber. As the name suggests, soluble fiber dissolves in water to form a soft, gooey liquid or gel that can be fermented by the bacteria in the gut and absorbed by the body. Soluble fiber is found in oatmeal, pulses such as lentils, fruits such as oranges and bananas and some vegetables, especially corn and green, leafy vegetables.

Insoluble fiber cannot be digested by the body and passes through unchanged. It is found in cereal-based foods such as whole-wheat bread, whole-wheat pasta, brown rice, whole-wheat and bran breakfast cereals and the skins of some fruits and vegetables.

Both soluble and insoluble fiber are important to maintain a healthy digestive system. Low intakes of dietary fiber are associated with an increased risk of bowel disease as well as disorders such as constipation. Fiber, particularly cereal (insoluble) fiber, helps to regulate bowel function and prevent intestinal disorders such as piles (hemorrhoids) and diverticular disease.

Dietary fiber is also thought to offer some protection against diseases such as colon cancer and is sometimes successful in treating irritable bowel syndrome. Research suggests that small amounts of soluble fiber are digested into the bloodstream, and this is thought to help to lower high cholesterol levels in the blood. It is believed that fiber reduces the rate at which carbohydrates are digested and transformed into blood sugar, a fact that has implications for diabetics.

It is very important to drink plenty of nonalcoholic fluids as part of a healthy diet—at least eight glasses a day (preferably water). This is especially true when the diet is high in fiber. Undigested fiber absorbs and holds fluid in the gut to form soft and bulky stools that move quickly and efficiently along the bowel. As already stated, water is the best beverage, but some fruit juices, milk (low-fat in the case of adults) and limited amounts of coffee and tea are all acceptable. If insufficient liquid is drunk, constipation may be the result.

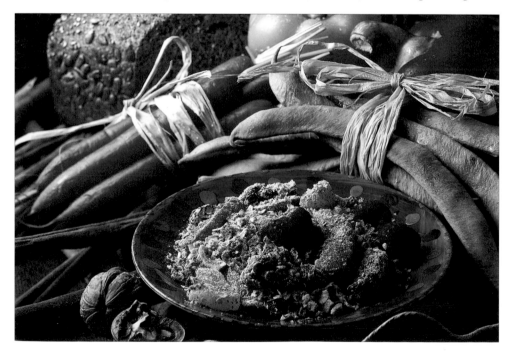

*Left: Increase your fiber intake at breakfast time by enjoying high-fiber muesli sprinkled over fresh fruit. The tastiest and healthiest muesli is homemade from oats, bran flakes, wheat germ, dried fruit, nuts and seeds.*

## INTRODUCING MORE FIBER

There are many simple ways of introducing fiber into your diet. Some years ago, it became fashionable to boost fiber by simply sprinkling bran on anything and everything, from breakfast cereals to stews and desserts. While wheat bran is a good source of fiber, simply adding it to your food is no substitute for getting fiber from food itself. Wheat bran can be an irritant; it is high in substances called phytates, which can interfere with the absorption of essential minerals such as iron, calcium and zinc.

It is important to obtain a mixture of both soluble and insoluble fiber from a variety of foods that are naturally good sources of fiber, rather than taking supplements. By choosing foods that are naturally high in fiber you will benefit from other important nutrients such as vitamins and minerals in those foods. For example, switching from white bread, pasta and rice to whole-wheat or whole-grain alternatives is an easy way of introducing more fiber into your diet, as is choosing a whole-wheat breakfast cereal or serving a baked potato with a meal.

Many foods that are higher in fiber also tend to be filling, bulky and relatively low in calories. Weight watchers and dieters who fill up on high-fiber, starchy foods like whole-grain cereals, bread, pasta and rice have less room for refined foods, which tend to be higher in fat and sugar.

Nowadays, many packaged foods are labeled with nutritional information, including the dietary fiber content. It is a good idea to get into the habit of reading the labels, not just for the amount of fiber, but also for the levels of other nutrients. Food charts listing the fiber content of everyday foods, are included in this book.

*Right: Whole-wheat bread is a good source of fiber and is full of flavor. It is available in a wide range of foods, from the traditional farmhouse loaf to rolls, muffins and pita bread.*

### FIBER BOOSTERS

Quick and easy ways of increasing the amount of fiber in the diet:
- Choose whole-wheat, whole-grain, high-fiber or brown bread for snacks, sandwiches and serving with meals. Look for whole-wheat pita bread, rolls, muffins, scones, buns, cookies, crackers and crispbreads, too. Add whole-wheat bread crumbs to stuffings, coatings and toppings.
- Choose whole-wheat flour rather than white flour and whole-wheat pasta instead of white pasta.
- Brown rice has more fiber than white rice and has a delicious, nutty taste. Try a medley of brown and wild rice.
- Select whole-wheat breakfast cereals that are naturally high in fiber rather than adding neat bran to cereals. Make your own high-fiber muesli by mixing oats, bran flakes, wheat germ, dried fruit, nuts and seeds. Serve topped with some fresh fruit.
- Use whole-wheat breakfast cereals and muesli in baking, for topping fruit crumble, as coatings and in cheesecake crust, meat loaves and burgers.
- Base a main course entirely on pulses rather than meat or fish; alternatively, replace some of the meat with cooked beans or lentils. Soups can be similarly extended, and fresh vegetables, such as carrots and potatoes, can be added.
- Wash but don't peel fruit and vegetables where possible. When making vegetable soups or sauces, leave the vegetables in chunks. If you must purée them, do not sieve the purée or you will lose much of the valuable fiber.
- Add grated root vegetables, such as potatoes or parsnips, to casseroles, lasagne, shepherd's pie and stews.
- Enjoy at least five portions of fresh vegetables or fruit every day on their own or in salads, lightly cooked or, ideally, raw.
- Snack on dried fruit, or use it in cakes, scones and muffins. Dried fruit salad is delicious.

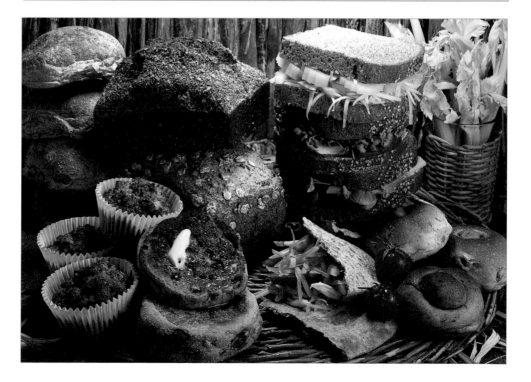

# PANTRY INGREDIENTS

Many simple, high-fiber ingredients are available in packages or cans. Keep your pantry stocked with the items in the list that follows, and increasing the fiber content of a snack or meal will always be easy.

### BREAKFAST CEREALS

A wide variety of breakfast cereals is available. Whole-wheat or whole-grain varieties are the best choice for fiber—preferably those that are also low in fat and sugar. Try using whole-wheat breakfast cereals when making homemade baked goods such as muesli bars and pancakes, for crumble toppings and cheesecake crusts, for coating foods, in tea breads and meat loaves or burgers.

### BROWN RICE

There are many varieties of brown rice available including long-grain, basmati, jasmine and risotto, as well as canned brown rice and boil-in-the-bag brown rice for convenience.

The flavor of brown rice is quite nutty and because the rice undergoes only minor milling, the bran layer is retained, making it higher in fiber, vitamins and minerals than white rice. Rice is also low in fat. Cooking time for brown rice is about 35 minutes, during which time it expands and increases by up to three times the volume. Allow at least $1/3$ cup uncooked rice per person.

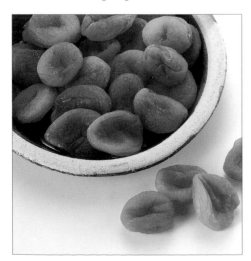

### CANNED BEANS AND OTHER PULSES

There are many kinds of canned pulses, such as beans, peas and lentils, available in shops and supermarkets. They include black-eyed beans, lima beans, pinto beans, chickpeas, flageolet beans, lentils, peas and red kidney beans. They are low in fat and high in protein, vitamins and minerals.

Add beans and other pulses to dishes such as salads, soups, pâtés and burgers, or try mashing cooked pulses to use as a basis for dips, served with vegetable crudités.

### DRIED BEANS AND OTHER PULSES

Dried pulses are very useful pantry items. When buying, choose dried pulses that are plump, bright and clear in color. Store in an airtight container and use within one year.

Many dried pulses need to be soaked in water before being cooked and should be boiled for a period, until tender. The older the beans are, the longer they will take to cook. Salt should be added only at the end of the cooking time; if added sooner, it will toughen the beans. Some beans, such as red kidney beans, contain a toxic substance known as hemaglutinin that can lead to acute gastroenteritis if it is not destroyed by adequate cooking. These beans should to be boiled vigorously for at least 10 minutes to destroy the hemaglutinin, then simmered until they are tender.

### DRIED FRUIT

Supermarkets, health-food stores and even corner shops stock a good selection of dried fruit including apples, apricots, bananas, currants, figs, kiwifruit, lychees, mangoes, papayas, peaches, pears, pineapple, prunes,

*Left: Dried apricots make a delicious snack between meals and are very high in fiber.*

raisins and golden raisins. They are very versatile and can be used in both sweet and savory dishes. Add dried fruit to your breakfast cereal, muesli or oatmeal, and use it in cake, scone, cookie and muffin recipes.

### NUTS

Nuts are a good source of dietary fiber and have many uses in a wide selection of sweet and savory dishes. They also make a tasty snack, but as they are high in fat and calories, eat them only in small quantities. Nuts yielding generous amounts of dietary fiber include almonds, brazil nuts, hazelnuts, peanuts, pecans, pistachios and walnuts.

Some nuts, such as almonds and hazelnuts, are also a good source of vitamin E. Add nuts to salads, cakes, cookies, desserts, stuffings, coatings and stir-fries. Nuts also make a good topping for a gratin and can be used as a garnish for savory dishes or a decoration for desserts.

### OATS AND OATMEAL

Oats and oatmeal are valuable sources of soluble fiber, which is absorbed into the body and is thought to help reduce high levels of blood cholesterol. Oats and oatmeal come in a variety of forms including porridge oats, quick-cook oats, jumbo oats, fine and medium oatmeal. Use oats in muesli and oatcake mixed with flour for breads and rolls, cakes and baked goods such as gingerbread and pancakes, and crumble toppings. Fine oatmeal also makes a good thickener for soups and sauces.

### SEEDS

Seeds such as sesame, sunflower and pumpkin are all good sources of dietary fiber. They can be eaten on their own as a snack or added to dishes such as salads, stir-fries, stuffings, cakes and baked goods, coatings, muesli, cookies and crackers. Seeds also contain vitamins and minerals but are high in fat and calories, so they should be eaten in small quantities.

## SPICES

Spices are invaluable items for the pantry; they can enhance and transform everyday dishes. Keep them in airtight, tinted-glass containers in a cool, dark cupboard. Ground spices should be used within six months and whole spices within a year, so it is wise to buy them in small quantities. Freshly ground spices provide the best flavor and aroma; it is well-worth investing in a small mortar and pestle so that you can grind your own.

## SUGARS AND HONEY

There is no calorific difference between white (refined) and brown (unrefined) sugar, but the flavors vary. Many of the recipes in this book use light brown sugar, but other sugars, such as superfine or dark brown, can be used instead.

Honey is also used in sweet and savory dishes. Honey is a little sweeter than sugar, so if you are substituting it for sugar you will probably need slightly less.

## WHEAT BRAN

Natural wheat bran is the hard outer layer or casing that surrounds the wheat grain. It is high in fiber. Other brans, such as rice bran, oat bran and soy bran, are also available, but wheat bran is the most common.

Bran is a useful ingredient and can be added to breads, muffins and cereals, but sprinkling bran on a dish is no substitute for getting fiber from food.

## WHOLE-WHEAT COOKIES AND CRACKERS

Whole-wheat cookies and high-fiber crackers make good pantry standbys for a healthy, high-fiber snack. Serve savory varieties with a selection of cheeses, or spread with butter or a low-fat spread. Crushed, sweet whole-wheat cookies are good for cheesecake crusts and crunchy toppings for fruity desserts.

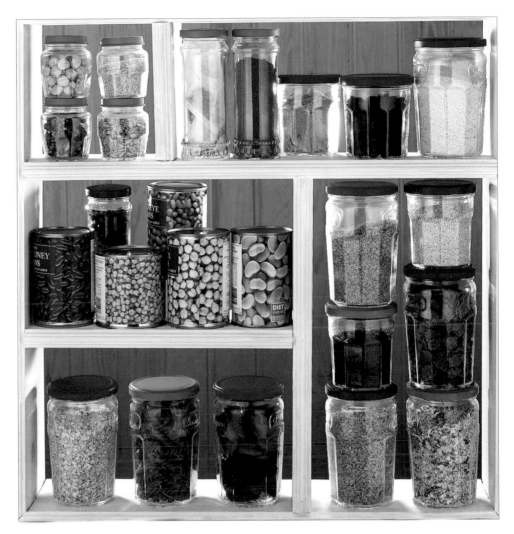

## WHOLE-WHEAT FLOUR

Whole-wheat flour is 100 percent flour that has been milled from the whole of the wheat grain. "Whole" means that the grain has not had the bran, vitamins and minerals refined out—in other words, it has had nothing added or removed, so it contains all the original nutrients and is by far the healthiest option.

Whole-wheat flour is coarser than white flour and available in several forms. It is very versatile and can be used in many dishes that traditionally specify white flour, including cakes, breads, pastry, cookies and crackers. It makes a good thickener for sauces and can be used to coat foods. A mixture of half whole-wheat and half white flour can be used in recipes where a lighter flour is required.

*Above: It is always worth keeping a useful selection of basic items in your pantry, including dried as well as canned ingredients.*

## WHOLE-WHEAT PASTA

Dried whole-wheat pasta is a good source of dietary fiber and carbohydrate. It is also low in fat and contains some B vitamins. It is an essential pantry item and a great basis for many quick and easy, nutritious meals. Pasta is very versatile and can be used in many dishes including salads, casseroles and filled pasta, which can be topped with low-fat sauces. Allow 1–2 cups pasta per serving for a main course and 1/2–1 cup per person for an appetizer. Dried whole-wheat pasta cooks in about 12 minutes.

# FRESH FOODS AND INGREDIENTS

Fresh vegetables and fruit play a vitally important part in a high-fiber diet. They are particularly wholesome if eaten raw and unpeeled. Whole-wheat bread and other baked goods are also excellent sources of fiber, as well as whole-wheat pastas and rice.

## FRESH BEANS AND OTHER LEGUMES

There are many varieties of fresh beans and legumes available including peas, fava beans and green beans, and more unusual ones such as fresh flageolet beans and lima beans. Fresh corn on the cob and baby corn are also popular.

All are good sources of dietary fiber and contain other nutrients including vitamins and minerals. Beans and legumes (known as pulses when dried) are very versatile and can be used in many dishes including salads, stir-fries, casseroles, pasta sauces, soups and curries. Some varieties, such as sugar-snap peas and snow peas, can be eaten either raw or cooked.

## FRESH FRUIT

Fresh fruit plays an important part in a healthy, balanced, high-fiber diet. Choose fruits that contain useful amounts of fiber such as apples, pears, bananas, oranges and peaches or berries such as raspberries, blackberries and gooseberries, not forgetting some more exotic fruits, including guavas and mangoes.

Fruits are very versatile and can be enjoyed raw or cooked, on their own or as part of a recipe. They are also good sources of vitamins and minerals. Avoid peeling them, when possible, for maximum nutrition.

## FRESH HERBS

In cooking, herbs are used mainly for their flavoring and seasoning properties, as well as for adding color and texture. Simply adding a single herb or a combination of herbs can transform everyday dishes into delicious meals. Herbs are also very low in fat and calories and some, such as parsley, provide a useful balance of vitamins and minerals.

## FRESH VEGETABLES

Fresh vegetables, like fresh fruit, play an important part in a healthy, balanced diet. We are advised to eat at least five portions of fruit and vegetables each day. Vegetables are nutritious and are valuable sources of vitamins and minerals, some being especially rich in vitamins A, C and E. Vegetables also contain some dietary fiber; those that are particularly good sources include broccoli, Brussels sprouts, cabbage, carrots, fennel, okra, parsnips, spinach and corn.

## POTATOES

Potatoes are among the most commonly eaten vegetables in the world and are valuable in terms of nutrition. They are high in carbohydrate, low in fat and contain some vitamin C and dietary fiber. Potatoes contain more dietary fiber when eaten unpeeled. Wash old and new potatoes thoroughly and cook them with their skins on—baked, boiled or roasted. Try mashed potatoes (with their skins left on, of course!) as a topping on savory pies and casseroles. Use skim milk, fromage frais, reduced-fat hard cheese or herbs to add flavor. For roast potatoes use only a small amount of oil, and if you must make french fries, leave the skins on and cut the fries thickly, using a knife.

## WHOLE-WHEAT BAKED GOODS AND BREAD

Whole-wheat pita breads, scones, muffins and tea cakes make good, high-fiber snacks or treats. Choose whole-wheat or whole-grain varieties whenever possible.

Bread is available in many varieties and is a good source of carbohydrate as well as being low in fat. It also contains some calcium, iron and B vitamins, and whole-wheat varieties are high in fiber.

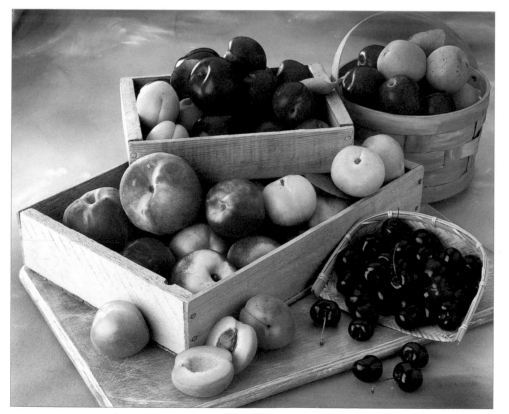

*Left: Eat fresh fruit regularly, as it contains vitamin C as well as being high in fiber.*

# HIGH FIBER MEAL PLANNER

In the at-a-glance guide that follows, six typical sweet and savory dishes are contrasted with similar dishes that have been altered slightly to increase their fiber content. (The full recipes are given in this book). The changes are simple, but the results are significant. Each dish has been analyzed to reveal the dietary fiber content of a typical serving, and to illustrate how easy it is to boost your intake of fiber by making only minimal changes to your diet. This will help you to choose the right ingredients when you prepare your own recipes.

---

**FRESH TOMATO SOUP *VERSUS* FRESH TOMATO, LENTIL AND ONION SOUP**

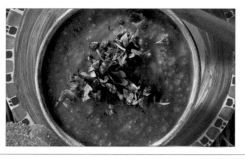

The dietary fiber content of an average portion of fresh tomato soup is 3.09 grams. Use fewer tomatoes and add onions and lentils; however, and the dietary fiber content per portion rises a little to 4.27grams.

---

**CHEESE AND TOMATO PIZZA WITH WHITE SCONE CRUST *VERSUS* ZUCCHINI, CORN AND PLUM TOMATO PIZZA WITH WHOLE-WHEAT CRUST**

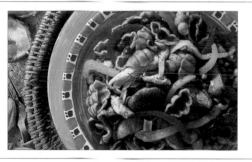

With a white scone crust, an average slice of cheese and tomato pizza has a dietary fiber content of 1.99 grams. Use whole-wheat flour for the crust and add mushrooms, zucchini, onion and corn to the topping, and the dietary fiber content rises to 4.93grams.

---

**WHITE PASTA SALAD WITH BELL PEPPERS AND MUSHROOMS *VERSUS* ROASTED BELL PEPPER AND WILD MUSHROOM PASTA SALAD**

The dietary fiber content of an average portion of pasta salad with peppers and mushrooms is 5.82 grams. To boost this to 9.37 grams, use whole-wheat pasta instead of white pasta and golden raisins instead of cherry tomatoes.

---

**ORDINARY COLESLAW *VERSUS* CARROT, RAISIN AND APRICOT COLESLAW**

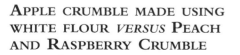

An average portion of ordinary coleslaw has a dietary fiber content of 2.92 grams. If the quantity of cabbage is reduced slightly and celery, raisins and dried apricots are added, this rises to 4.25 grams.

---

**APPLE CRUMBLE MADE USING WHITE FLOUR *VERSUS* PEACH AND RASPBERRY CRUMBLE**

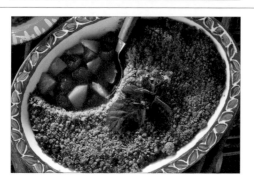

The dietary fiber content of an average portion of apple crumble is 3.86 grams. However, if a mixture of whole-wheat flour and oatmeal is used in place of white flour to make the crumble topping, and peaches and raspberries replace apples for the base, this will rise to 5.22 grams.

# High Fiber Food Charts

The following tables are an at-a-glance guide to the dietary fiber content of a range of commonly eaten foods. The figures show the amount of fiber per 3³/4 ounces, unless otherwise stated. For cereals, a 1¾ ounces serving size is also given.

| Beans, Peas and Lentils | Fiber (g) |
|---|---|
| baked beans in tomato sauce | 3.7 |
| fava beans, boiled | 6.5 |
| lima beans, canned | 4.6 |
| chickpeas, canned | 4.1 |
| green beans, boiled | 4.1 |
| lentils, brown and green, boiled | 3.8 |
| lentils, red split, boiled | 1.9 |
| peas, boiled | 5.1 |
| red kidney beans, canned | 6.2 |
| navy beans, dry | 12.0 |
| snow peas, boiled | 2.2 |

| Cookies | Fiber (g) |
|---|---|
| cream cracker | 2.2 |
| cream cracker (each) | 0.2 |
| crispbread, rye | 11.7 |
| crispbread, rye (each) | 1.2 |
| crispbread, high fiber | 17.9 |
| crispbread, high fiber (each) | 1.8 |
| digestive, plain | 2.2 |
| digestive, plain (each) | 0.3 |
| oatcake | 5.9 |
| oatcake (each) | 0.8 |
| shortbread finger | 1.9 |
| shortbread finger (each) | 0.2 |

| Breads | Fiber (g) |
|---|---|
| brown bread | 3.5 |
| brown bread (1 medium slice) | 1.3 |
| white pita bread | 2.2 |
| white pita bread (1 medium pitta) | 1.4 |
| whole-wheat pita bread | 6.4 |
| whole-wheat pita (1 medium pitta) | 4.1 |
| rye bread | 4.4 |
| rye bread (1 average slice) | 1.1 |
| white bread | 1.5 |
| white bread (1 medium slice) | 0.5 |
| white bread with added fiber | 3.1 |
| white bread with added fiber (1 medium slice) | 1.1 |
| whole-wheat bread | 5.8 |
| whole-wheat bread (1 medium slice) | 2.1 |

The information presented in these tables has been compiled from McCance and Widdowson's *The Composition of Foods*, 5th edition and relevant supplements. Data are reproduced with the kind permission of the Royal Society of Chemistry and the Controller of Her Majesty's Stationery Office.

| Breakfast Cereals | Fiber (g) |
|---|---|
| All-bran | 24.5 |
| All-bran (1¾ oz serving) | 7.4 |
| Branflakes | 13.0 |
| Branflakes (1¾ oz serving) | 3.9 |
| Cheerios | 1.5 |
| Cheerios (1¾ oz serving) | 0.8 |
| Cornflakes | 0.9 |
| Cornflakes (1¾ oz serving) | 0.3 |
| Frosted Flakes | 0.8 |
| Frosted Flakes (1¾ oz serving) | 0.4 |
| Fruit 'n' fiber | 7.0 |
| Fruit 'n' fiber (1¾ oz serving) | 2.1 |
| muesli—Swiss style | 6.4 |
| muesli—Swiss style (1¾ oz serving) | 1.9 |
| muesli—no added sugar | 7.6 |
| muesli—no added sugar (1¾ oz) | 2.3 |
| oatmeal | 0.8 |
| oatmeal (1¾ oz serving) | 0.2 |
| Puffed Wheat | 5.6 |
| Puffed Wheat (1¾ oz serving) | 1.7 |
| Rice Crispies | 0.7 |
| Rice Crispies (1¾ oz serving) | 0.2 |
| Shredded Wheat | 9.8 |
| Shredded Wheat (1¾ oz serving) | 2.9 |
| Raisin Bran | 10.0 |
| Raisin Bran (1¾ oz serving) | 3.0 |

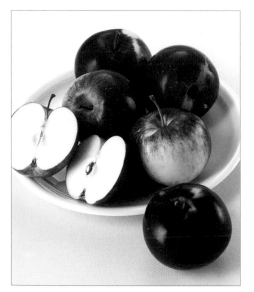

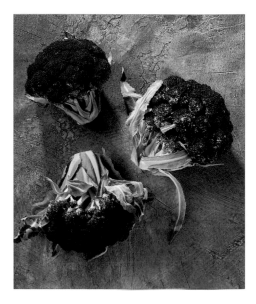

*Left: Apples and other fresh fruit make a healthy snack at any time of the day. If possible, increase your fiber intake by eating the skins of all fruit with edible skins.*

*Right: Broccoli or other fresh vegetables should be eaten every day. Consuming them raw rather than cooked is a much more healthy way of eating them.*

| BAKED GOODS | FIBER (G) |
|---|---|
| fruit cake, rich | 1.7 |
| fruit cake, rich (per slice) | 1.2 |
| fruit cake, whole-wheat | 2.4 |
| fruit cake, whole-wheat (per slice) | 1.7 |
| sponge cake | 0.9 |
| sponge cake (per slice) | 0.5 |
| muffin, plain | 2.0 |
| muffin, plain (each) | 1.4 |
| muffin, bran | 7.7 |
| muffin, bran (each) | 5.4 |
| scone, plain | 1.9 |
| scone, plain (each) | 0.9 |
| scone, whole-wheat | 5.2 |
| scone, whole-wheat (each) | 2.6 |

| FLOURS AND GRAINS | FIBER (G) |
|---|---|
| wheat bran | 36.4 |
| oatmeal | 6.8 |
| porridge oats | 7.0 |
| wheat flour, brown | 6.4 |
| wheat flour, white | 3.1 |
| wheat flour, whole-wheat | 9.0 |
| wheat germ | 15.6 |
| brown rice, boiled | 0.8 |
| white rice, boiled | 0.1 |
| white spaghetti, boiled | 1.2 |
| whole-wheat spaghetti, boiled | 3.5 |

| FRUIT | FIBER (G) |
|---|---|
| (Figures given are for raw fruit unless otherwise stated) | |
| apple, eating | 1.8 |
| apple, eating (each) | 1.8 |
| apricots, dried | 6.3 |
| avocado | 3.4 |
| banana | 1.1 |
| banana (each) | 1.1 |
| blackberries | 3.1 |
| dates, dried | 3.4 |
| figs, dried | 6.9 |
| golden raisins | 2.0 |
| blueberries | 2.0 |
| grapefruit | 1.3 |
| grapefruit (half) | 1.0 |
| guava | 3.7 |
| kiwifruit | 1.9 |
| kiwifruit (each) | 1.1 |
| mango | 2.6 |
| orange | 1.7 |
| orange (each) | 2.7 |
| passion fruit | 3.3 |
| passion fruit (each) | 0.5 |
| peach | 1.5 |
| peach (each) | 1.7 |
| peaches, dried | 7.3 |
| pear | 2.2 |
| pear (each) | 3.3 |
| pears, dried | 8.3 |
| pineapple | 1.2 |
| pineapple, dried | 8.1 |
| prunes | 5.7 |
| raisins | 2.0 |
| raspberries | 2.5 |

| NUTS AND SEEDS | FIBER (G) |
|---|---|
| almonds | 7.4 |
| brazil nuts | 4.3 |
| chestnuts | 4.1 |
| dried coconut | 13.7 |
| hazelnuts | 6.5 |
| peanuts | 6.2 |
| pecans | 4.7 |
| pistachios | 6.1 |
| pumpkin seeds | 5.3 |
| sesame seeds | 7.9 |
| sunflower seeds | 6.0 |
| walnuts | 3.5 |

| PASTRY | FIBER (G) |
|---|---|
| shortcrust, cooked | 2.2 |
| whole-wheat shortcrust, cooked | 6.3 |

| VEGETABLES | FIBER (G) |
|---|---|
| broccoli, boiled | 2.3 |
| Brussels sprouts, boiled | 3.1 |
| cabbage, raw | 2.4 |
| cabbage, boiled | 1.8 |
| carrots, raw | 2.4 |
| carrots, boiled | 2.5 |
| celeriac, boiled | 3.2 |
| collard greens, boiled | 2.6 |
| corn kernels, canned | 1.9 |
| fennel, boiled | 2.3 |
| leeks, boiled | 1.7 |
| mushrooms, canned | 2.0 |
| okra, boiled | 3.6 |
| onions, raw | 1.4 |
| parsnips, boiled | 4.7 |
| potatoes, baked, flesh and skin | 2.7 |
| potatoes, boiled | 1.2 |
| spinach, raw | 2.1 |
| spinach, boiled | 2.1 |
| squash, baked | 2.1 |
| sweet potatoes, boiled | 2.3 |
| turnip, boiled | 1.4 |

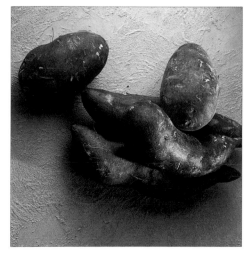

*Left: Sweet potatoes are rich in fiber and vitamins and do not take as long as ordinary potatoes to cook. Scrub them clean and bake in a hot oven in their skins for 10–15 minutes.*

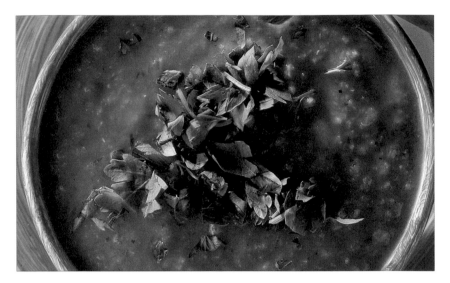

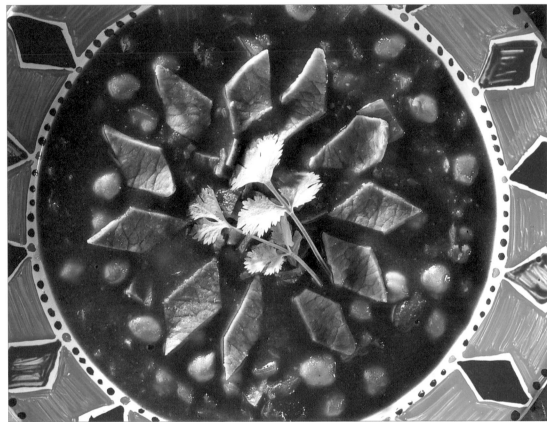

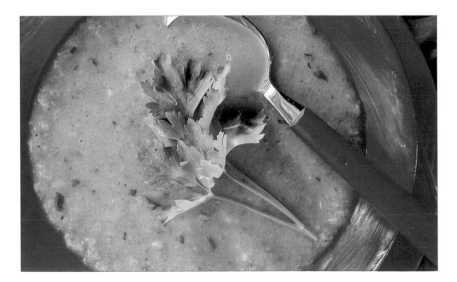

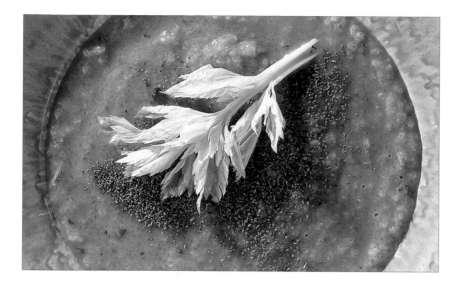

# SOUPS AND APPETIZERS

*For simple soups that are full of fiber, make the most of chickpeas, beans and lentils, alone or with fresh vegetables such as carrots, onions and leeks. Spicy Chickpea and Bacon Soup is a sure winner or, for vegetarians, go green with the very wholesome Pea, Leek and Broccoli Soup. Appetizers include a delicious dip with lima beans as the prime ingredient, which is accompanied by crunchy vegetable crudités, while kidney beans combine with fresh mushrooms to make an unforgettable pâté. Vegetables are worthy of a starring role, served on their own as in Vegetables Provençal or with chicken in a wonderful, warm salad. Serve soups and appetizers with whole-wheat bread to boost the fiber content of your meal still further.*

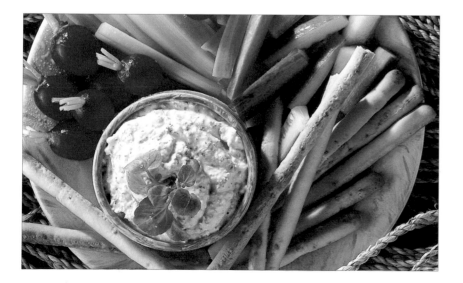

# Spicy Chickpea and Bacon Soup

This is a tasty mixture of chickpeas and bacon, flavored with a subtle mix of spices.

## INGREDIENTS

*Serves 4–6*
2 teaspoons sunflower oil
1 onion, chopped
2 garlic cloves, crushed
1 teaspoon each garam masala,
   ground coriander, ground cumin
   and ground turmeric
½ teaspoon hot chili powder
2 tablespoons whole-wheat flour
2½ cups vegetable stock
14-ounce can chopped tomatoes
14-ounce can chickpeas, rinsed
   and drained
6 strips lean smoked Canadian bacon
salt and ground black pepper
cilantro sprigs, to garnish

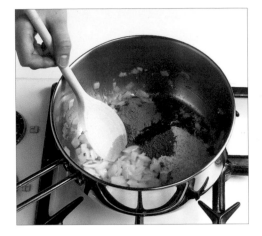

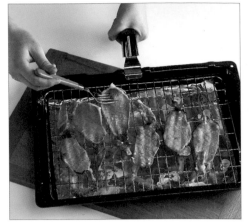

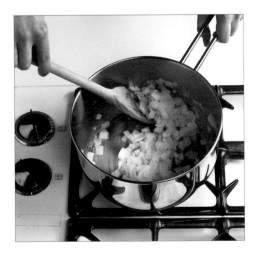

*1* Heat the oil in a large saucepan. Add the onion and garlic and cook for 5 minutes, stirring occasionally so that the mixture does not burn.

*2* Add the spices and flour and cook for 1 minute, stirring.

*5* Meanwhile, cook the bacon for about 2–3 minutes on each side.

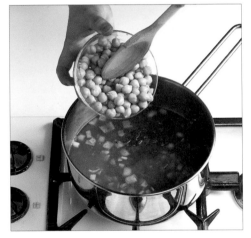

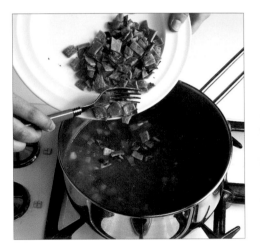

*3* Gradually add the stock, stirring constantly, and then add the tomatoes and chickpeas.

*6* Dice the bacon, cutting and reserving a few diamond-shaped pieces for garnishing. Stir the diced pieces into the hot soup. Season to taste, reheat gently until piping hot and ladle the soup into bowls. Garnish each bowl with a cilantro sprig and the reserved bacon. Serve immediately.

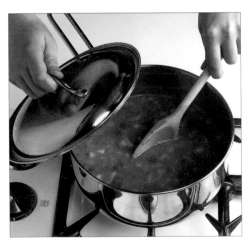

*4* Bring to a boil, stirring, then cover and simmer for 25 minutes, stirring occasionally.

--- VARIATION ---

Use other canned beans such as red kidney beans or flageolet beans in place of the chickpeas for a different flavor.

--- NUTRITION NOTES ---

| Per portion: | |
| --- | --- |
| Energy | 207kcals |
| Protein | 15.56g |
| Fat | 7.28g |
| Saturated fat | 1.43g |
| Carbohydrate | 22.40g |
| Fiber | 4.82g |
| Added sugar | 0.02g |
| Sodium | 1.17g |

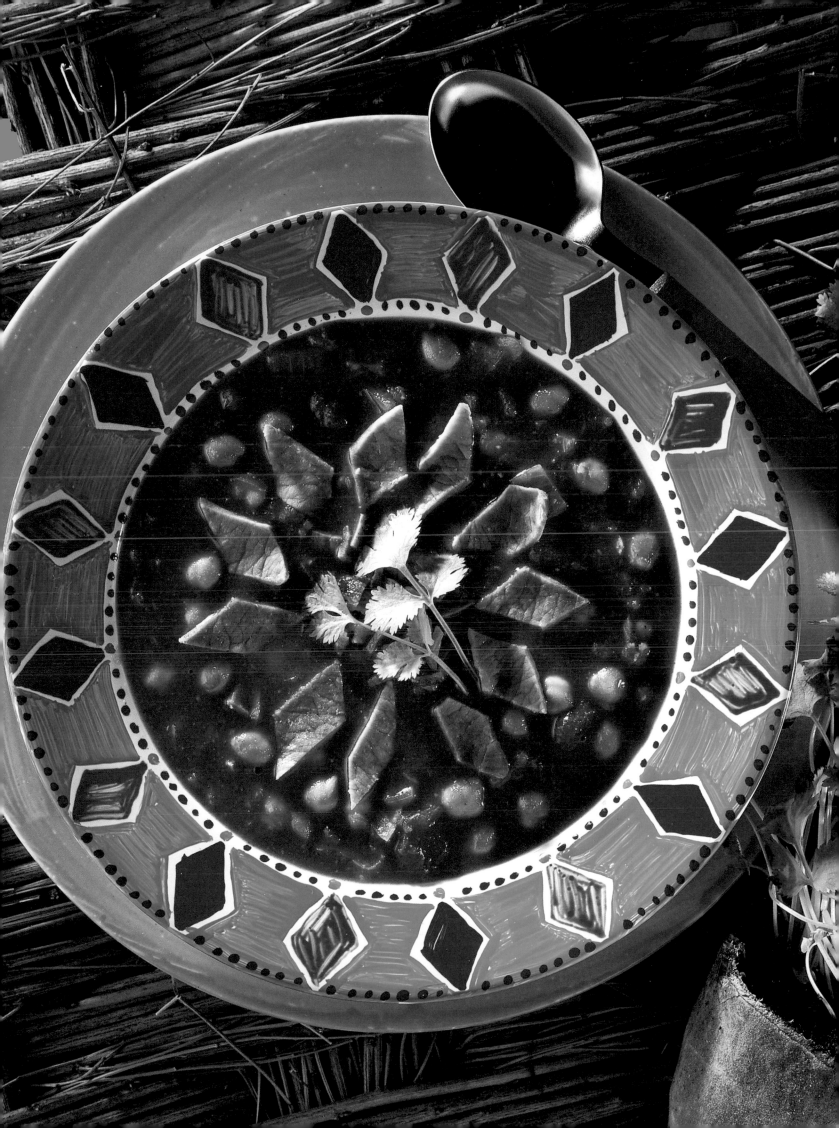

# Fresh Tomato, Lentil and Onion Soup

This delicious, wholesome soup is ideal served with thick slices of whole-wheat bread.

## INGREDIENTS

*Serves 4–6*

2 teaspoons sunflower oil
1 large onion, chopped
2 celery stalks, chopped
¾ cup split red lentils
2 large tomatoes, skinned and
    roughly chopped
3¾ cups vegetable stock
2 teaspoons dried herbes
    de Provence
salt and ground black pepper
chopped fresh parsley, to garnish

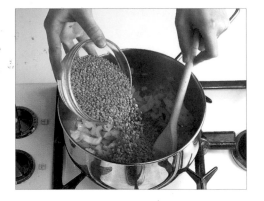

*1* Heat the oil in a large saucepan. Add the onion and celery and cook for 5 minutes, stirring occasionally. Add the lentils and cook for 1 minute.

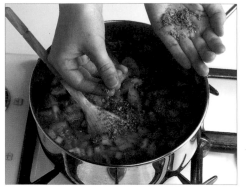

*2* Stir in the tomatoes, stock, herbs and seasoning. Cover, bring to a boil and simmer for about 20 minutes, stirring occasionally.

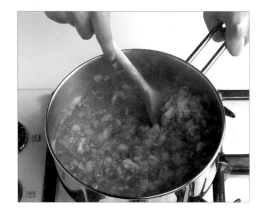

*3* When the lentils are cooked and tender, remove the soup from heat, and set aside to cool slightly.

*4* Purée in a blender or food processor until smooth. Adjust the seasoning, return to the saucepan and reheat gently until piping hot. Ladle into soup bowls and garnish each with chopped parsley.

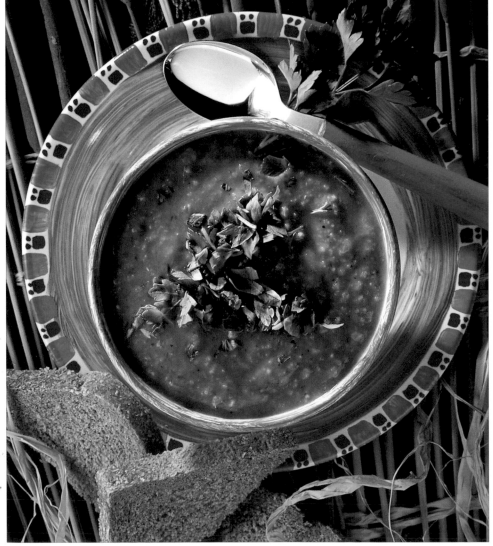

| NUTRITION NOTES | |
| --- | --- |
| Per portion: | |
| Energy | 202kcals |
| Protein | 12.40g |
| Fat | 3.07g |
| Saturated fat | 0.38g |
| Carbohydrate | 33.34g |
| Fiber | 4.27g |
| Added sugar | 0.04g |
| Sodium | 0.54g |

# Pea, Leek and Broccoli Soup

A nutritious soup, full of flavor and perfect for warming those chilly winter evenings.

## INGREDIENTS

*Serves 4–6*
1 onion, chopped
2 cups leeks, sliced
8 ounces unpeeled potatoes, diced
3¾ cups vegetable stock
1 bay leaf
8 ounces broccoli florets
1½ cups frozen peas
2–3 tablespoons chopped
   fresh parsley
salt and ground black pepper
parsley leaves, to garnish

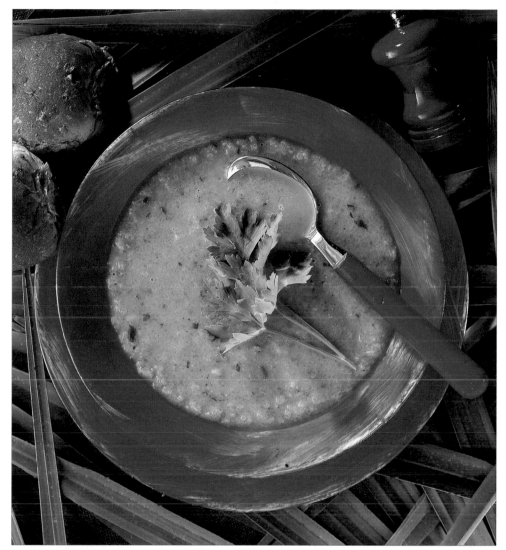

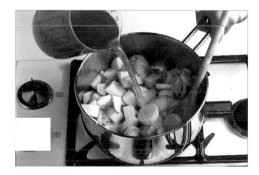

*1* Put the onion, leeks, potatoes, stock and bay leaf in a large saucepan and mix together. Cover, bring to a boil and simmer for 10 minutes, stirring.

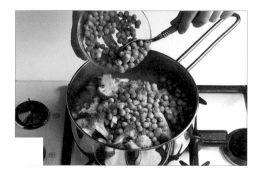

*2* Add the broccoli and peas, cover, return to a boil and simmer for another 10 minutes, stirring from time to time.

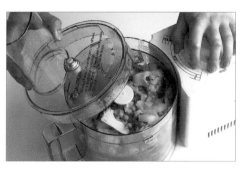

*3* Let cool slightly and remove and discard the bay leaf. Purée in a blender or food processor until smooth.

### COOK'S TIP

If you prefer, cut the vegetables finely and leave the cooked soup chunky rather than puréeing it.

*4* Add the chopped fresh parsley, season to taste and process again briefly. Return the soup to the saucepan and reheat gently until piping hot. Ladle into soup bowls and garnish with parsley leaves.

### NUTRITION NOTES

| Per portion: | |
| --- | --- |
| Energy | 125kcals |
| Protein | 8.11g |
| Fat | 1.92g |
| Saturated fat | 0.26g |
| Carbohydrate | 19.94g |
| Fiber | 6.31g |
| Added sugar | 0.04g |
| Sodium | 0.52g |

# Curried Celery Soup

A successful combination of flavors, this warming soup is excellent served with warm whole-wheat bread rolls or whole-wheat pita bread.

## INGREDIENTS

*Serves 4–6*
2 teaspoons olive oil
1 onion, chopped
1 leek, washed and sliced
1½ pounds celery, chopped
1 tablespoon medium or hot
  curry powder
8 ounces unpeeled potatoes,
  washed and diced
3¾ cups vegetable stock
1 bouquet garni
2 tablespoons chopped fresh
  mixed herbs
salt and ground black pepper
celery seeds and leaves, to garnish

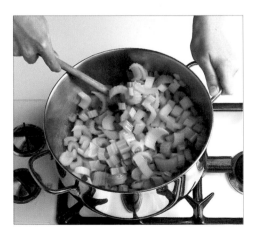

*1* Heat the oil in a large saucepan. Add the onion, leek and celery, cover and cook gently for 10 minutes, stirring occasionally.

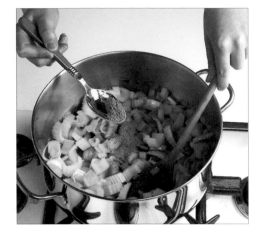

*2* Add the curry powder and cook for 2 minutes, stirring occasionally.

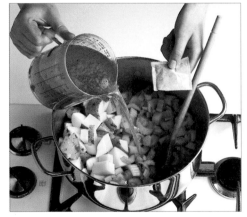

*3* Add the potatoes, stock and bouquet garni, cover, and bring to a boil. Simmer for 20 minutes, until the vegetables are tender.

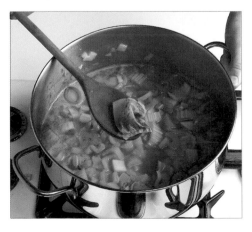

*4* Remove the saucepan from heat and discard the bouquet garni. Set the soup aside and allow it to cool slightly.

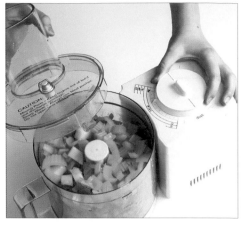

*5* Purée the soup in a blender or food processor until smooth.

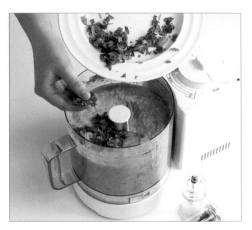

*6* Add the chopped fresh mixed herbs, season to taste and process again briefly. Return the soup to the saucepan and reheat gently until piping hot. Ladle into soup bowls and garnish each with a sprinkling of celery seeds and some celery leaves.

---

### VARIATION

For a tasty and sweeter change, use celeriac and sweet potatoes in place of celery and standard potatoes.

---

### NUTRITION NOTES

Per portion:

| | |
|---|---|
| Energy | 102kcals |
| Protein | 3.72g |
| Fat | 2.93g |
| Saturated fat | 0.25g |
| Carbohydrate | 16.11g |
| Fiber | 4.44g |
| Added sugar | 0.04g |
| Sodium | 0.62g |

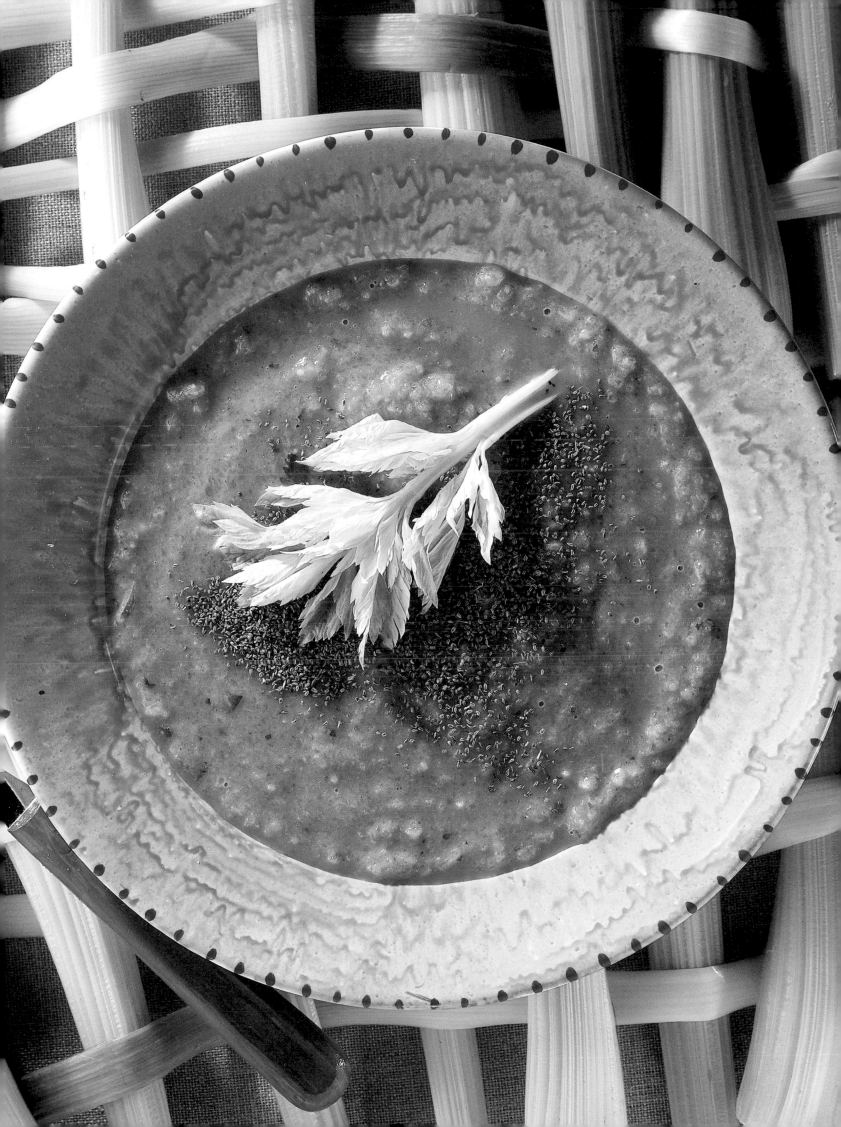

# Mushroom and Bean Pâté

Serve this unusual vegetarian pâté with whole-wheat bread or toast for an appetizer or a light suppertime snack. It also has the benefit of being very low in fat.

## INGREDIENTS

*Serves 12*

6 cups mushrooms, sliced
1 onion, chopped
2 garlic cloves, crushed
1 red bell pepper, seeded and diced
2 tablespoons vegetable stock
2 tablespoons dry white wine
14-ounce can red kidney beans,
   rinsed and drained
1 egg, beaten
1 cup fresh whole-wheat bread crumbs
1 tablespoon chopped fresh thyme
1 tablespoon chopped fresh rosemary
salt and ground black pepper
lettuce and cherry tomatoes, to garnish

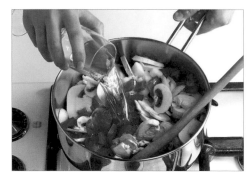

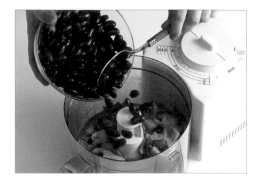

*1* Preheat the oven to 350°F. Lightly grease and line a nonstick 9 x 5 x 3-inch loaf pan. Put the mushrooms, onion, garlic, red pepper, stock and wine in a saucepan. Cover and cook for 10 minutes. Stir a little.

*2* Set aside to cool slightly, then purée the mixture with the kidney beans in a blender or food processor until smooth.

*3* Transfer the mixture to a bowl, add the egg, bread crumbs and herbs and mix thoroughly. Season to taste.

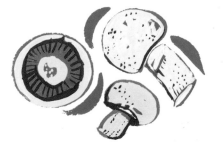

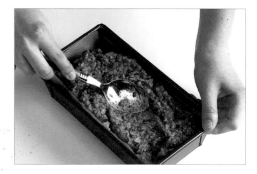

*4* Spoon into the prepared pan and level the surface. Bake for 45–60 minutes, until lightly set and browned on top. Place on a wire rack and allow the pâté to cool completely in the pan. Once cool, cover and refrigerate for several hours. Turn out of the pan and serve in slices. Garnish with lettuce and cherry tomatoes.

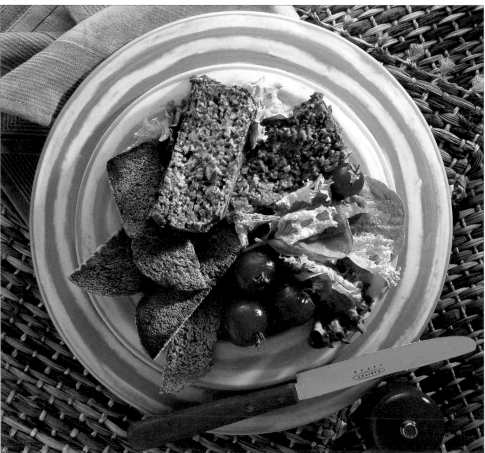

| — NUTRITION NOTES — | |
| --- | --- |
| Per portion: | |
| Energy | 53kcals |
| Protein | 3.42g |
| Fat | 1.04g |
| Saturated fat | 0.26g |
| Carbohydrate | 7.65g |
| Fiber | 2.33g |
| Added sugar | 0.00g |
| Sodium | 0.11g |

# Lima Bean, Watercress and Herb Dip

A refreshing dip that is especially good served with fresh vegetable crudités and breadsticks or even whole-wheat pita.

## INGREDIENTS

*Serves 4–6*

1 cup plain cottage cheese
14-ounce can lima beans, rinsed
   and drained
1 bunch scallions, chopped
2 ounces watercress, chopped
¼ cup reduced-calorie mayonnaise
3 tablespoons chopped fresh
   mixed herbs
salt and ground black pepper
watercress sprigs, to garnish
vegetable crudités and breadsticks,
   to serve

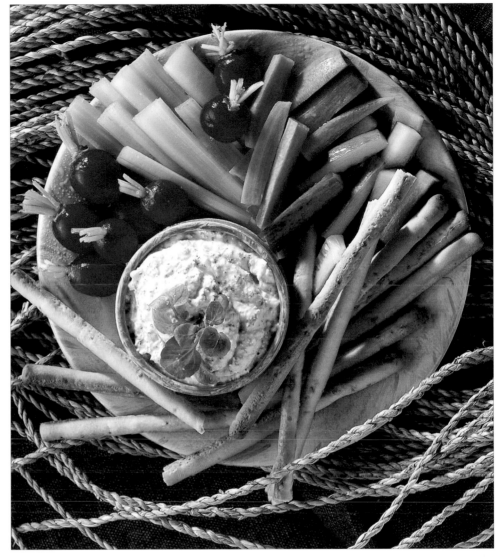

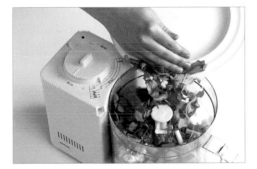

*1* Put the cottage cheese, beans, scallions, watercress, mayonnaise and herbs in a blender or food processor, and blend together until almost smooth.

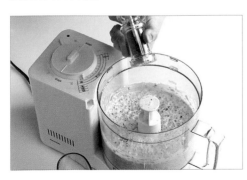

*2* Add seasoning and spoon the mixture carefully into a bowl. Stir well.

*3* Cover and chill for several hours before serving.

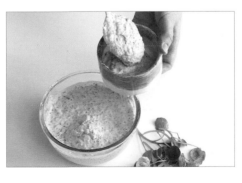

*4* Transfer to a serving dish (or individual dishes), and garnish with watercress sprigs. Serve with vegetable crudités and breadsticks.

---

NUTRITION NOTES

Per portion:

| | |
|---|---|
| Energy | 155kcals |
| Protein | 12.45g |
| Fat | 6.98g |
| Saturated fat | 2.04g |
| Carbohydrate | 11.25g |
| Fiber | 3.49g |
| Added sugar | 0.38g |
| Sodium | 0.63g |

---

VARIATION

Try using other canned pulses such as cannellini beans or chickpeas in place of the lima beans.

# Vegetables Provençal

The sunshine flavors of the Mediterranean are presented in this delicious vegetable dish, ideal for an appetizer or lunchtime snack served with fresh, crusty whole-wheat bread. It is an excellent dish for vegetarians.

## INGREDIENTS

*Serves 6*

1 onion, sliced
2 leeks, sliced
2 garlic cloves, crushed
1 red bell pepper, seeded and sliced
1 green bell pepper, seeded and sliced
1 yellow bell pepper, seeded and sliced
12 ounces zucchini, sliced
3 cups mushrooms, sliced
14-ounce can chopped tomatoes
2 tablespoons ruby port
2 tablespoons tomato paste
1 tablespoon ketchup
14-ounce can chickpeas
1 cup pitted black olives
3 tablespoons chopped fresh
    mixed herbs
salt and ground black pepper
chopped fresh mixed herbs,
    to garnish

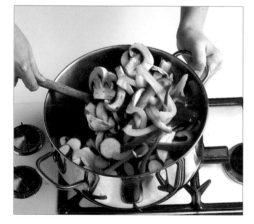

*1* Put the onion, leeks, garlic, peppers, zucchini and mushrooms into a large saucepan.

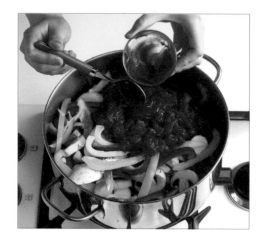

*2* Add the chopped tomatoes, port, tomato paste and ketchup, and mix well.

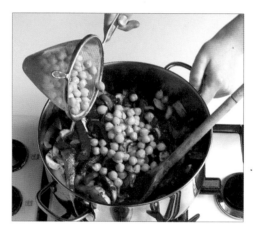

*3* Rinse and drain the chickpeas, and add to the pan.

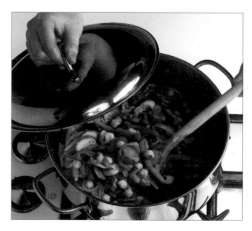

*4* Cover, bring to a boil and simmer gently for 20–30 minutes, until the vegetables are cooked and tender but not overcooked. Stir carefully from time to time.

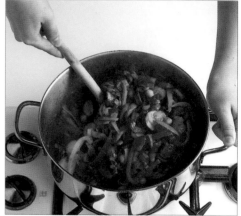

*5* Remove the lid and increase the heat slightly for the last 10 minutes of the cooking time to thicken the sauce, if desired.

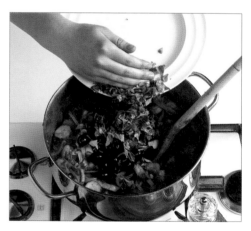

*6* Stir in the black olives, chopped fresh mixed herbs and seasoning. Serve the vegetables either hot or cold, garnished with additional chopped fresh mixed herbs.

| NUTRITION NOTES | |
| --- | --- |
| Per portion: | |
| Energy | 155kcals |
| Protein | 8.26g |
| Fat | 4.56g |
| Saturated fat | 0.67g |
| Carbohydrate | 20.19g |
| Fiber | 6.98g |
| Added sugar | 0.52g |
| Sodium | 0.62g |

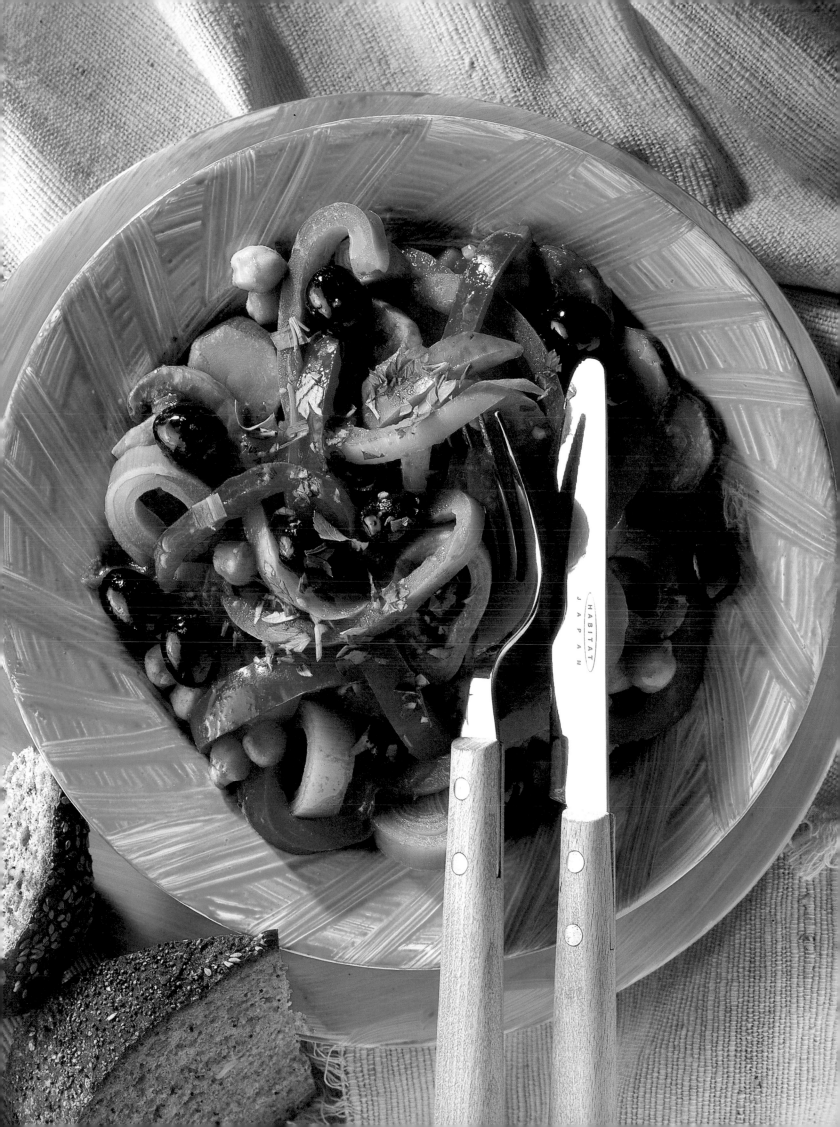

# Warm Chicken Salad with Shallots and Snow Peas

Succulent cooked chicken pieces are combined with vegetables in a light chili dressing.

**INGREDIENTS**

*Serves 6*

2 ounces mixed salad greens
2 ounces baby spinach leaves
2 ounces watercress
2 tablespoons chili sauce
2 tablespoons dry sherry
1 tablespoon light soy sauce
1 tablespoon ketchup
2 teaspoons olive oil
8 shallots, finely chopped
1 garlic clove, crushed
12 ounces skinless, boneless
  chicken breast, cut into thin strips
1 red bell pepper, seeded and sliced
6 ounces snow peas, trimmed
14-ounce can baby corn,
  drained and halved
10-ounce can brown rice
salt and ground black pepper
parsley sprig, to garnish

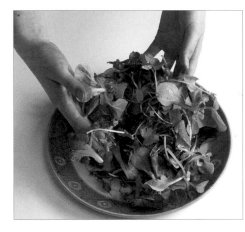

*1* Arrange the mixed salad greens, tearing up any large ones and the spinach leaves on a serving dish. Add the watercress and toss to mix.

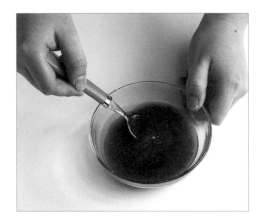

*2* In a small bowl, mix together the chili sauce, sherry, soy sauce and ketchup, and set aside.

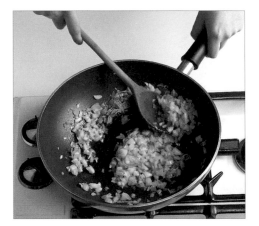

*3* Heat the oil in a large, nonstick frying pan or wok. Add the shallots and garlic, and stir-fry over medium heat for 1 minute.

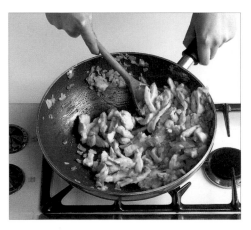

*4* Add the sliced chicken breast to the pan and stir-fry for another 4–5 minutes, until the chicken pieces are nearly cooked.

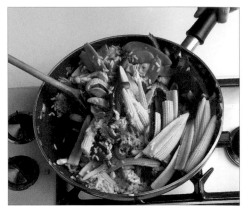

*5* Add the red pepper, snow peas, corn and rice, and stir-fry for 2–3 minutes.

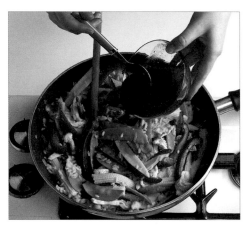

*6* Pour in the chili sauce mixture and stir-fry for 2–3 minutes, until hot and bubbling. Season to taste. Spoon the chicken mixture over the salad greens, toss together to mix and serve immediately, garnished with a sprig of parsley.

---

**VARIATION**

Use other kinds of lean meat—such as turkey breast or rindless bacon—in place of the chicken breast.

---

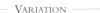

— NUTRITION NOTES —

Per portion:

| | |
|---|---|
| Energy | 188kcals |
| Protein | 19.22g |
| Fat | 2.81g |
| Saturated fat | 0.52g |
| Carbohydrate | 21.39g |
| Fiber | 3.07g |
| Added sugar | 0.71g |
| Sodium | 1.07g |

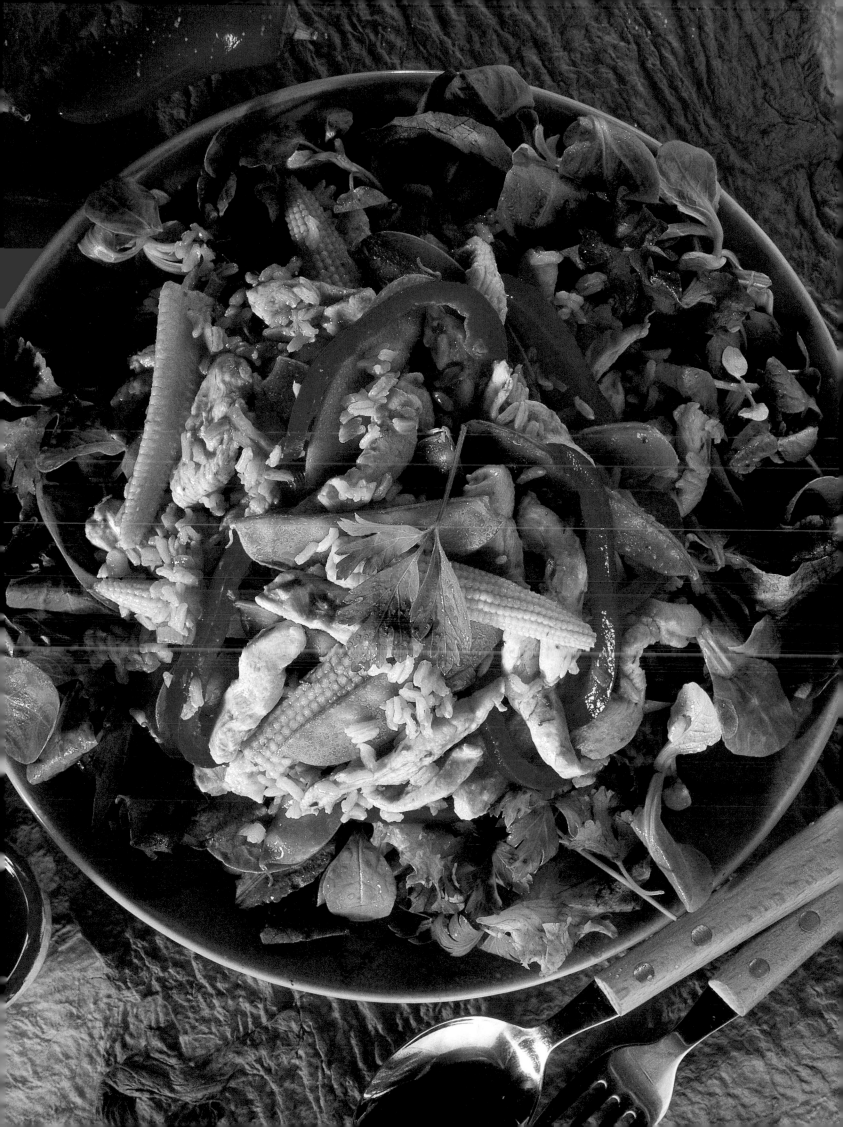

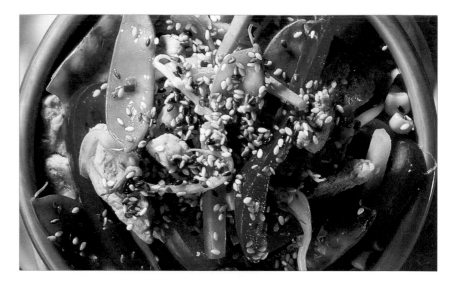

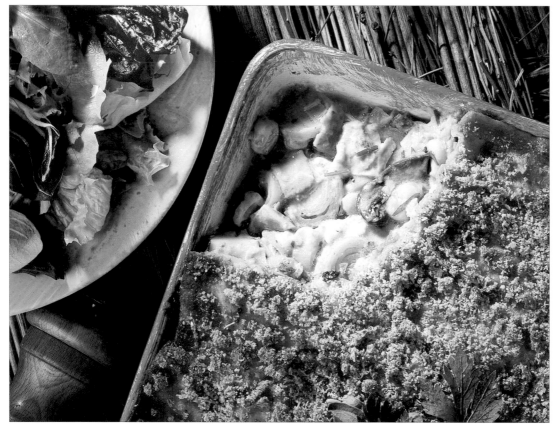

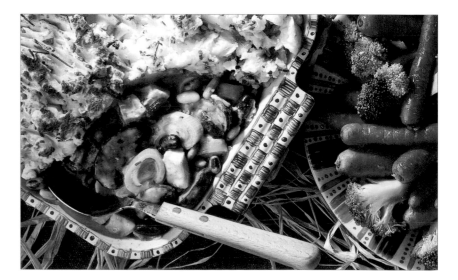

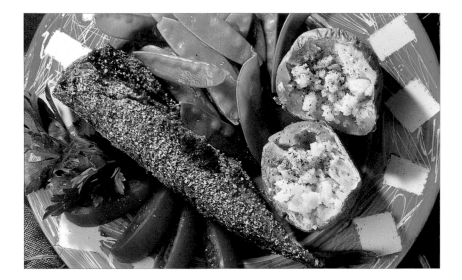

# MEAT, FISH AND POULTRY DISHES

*Increasing the fiber content of a meat, fish or poultry dish is simplicity itself.
All you need to do is add plenty of vegetables, which will also improve the
color, texture and flavor, or mix the meat with grains, pulses or pasta. This
not only serves as a cost-cutting exercise, making the main ingredient go
further, but also adds interest, as when couscous is combined with lamb in a
spicy stew, or green beans and pasta twists are partnered with smoked bacon to
make a salad. For a simple supper, toss mackerel in oatmeal and herbs, broil it
until tender and serve with tomatoes, snow peas and a baked potato, or make
a quick stir-fry using pieces of pork and vegetable chunks.*

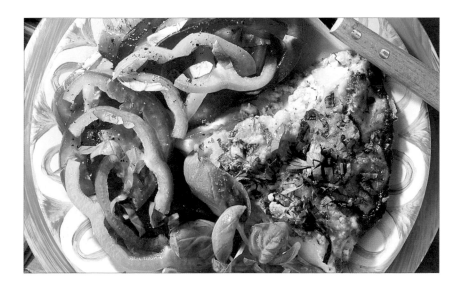

# Pork and Vegetable Stir-fry

A quick and easy stir-fry of pork and vegetables.

### INGREDIENTS

*Serves 4*

8-ounce can pineapple chunks
1 tablespoon cornstarch
2 tablespoons light soy sauce
1 tablespoon each dry sherry,
   brown sugar and wine vinegar
1 teaspoon five-spice powder
1-inch piece fresh ginger root
12 ounces lean pork tenderloin
2 teaspoons olive oil
1 red onion, sliced
1 garlic clove, crushed
1 fresh red chile, seeded and chopped
6 ounces carrots
1 red bell pepper, seeded and sliced
6 ounces snow peas
½ cup bean sprouts
7-ounce can corn kernels
2 tablespoons chopped fresh cilantro
salt and ground black pepper
1 tablespoon toasted sesame seeds,
   to garnish

1 Drain the pineapple, reserving the juice. In a small bowl, blend the cornstarch with the pineapple juice. Add the soy sauce, sherry, sugar, vinegar and spice. Stir to mix and set aside.

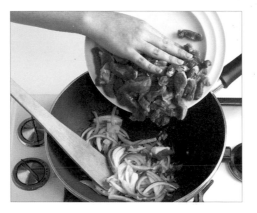

2 Peel and finely chop the ginger. Cut the pork into strips. Heat the oil in a large, nonstick frying pan or wok. Add the onion, garlic, chile and ginger, and stir-fry for 30 seconds. Then add the sliced pork and stir-fry for another 2–3 minutes.

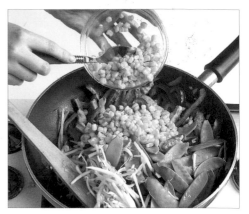

3 Cut the carrots into matchstick strips. Add to the wok with the red pepper and stir-fry for 2–3 minutes. Add the snow peas, bean sprouts and the drained corn, and stir-fry for 1–2 minutes.

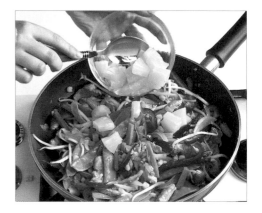

4 Pour in the sauce mixture and the reserved pineapple and stir-fry, until the sauce thickens. Reduce the heat and stir-fry for another 1–2 minutes. Stir in the cilantro and season to taste. Sprinkle with sesame seeds and serve immediately.

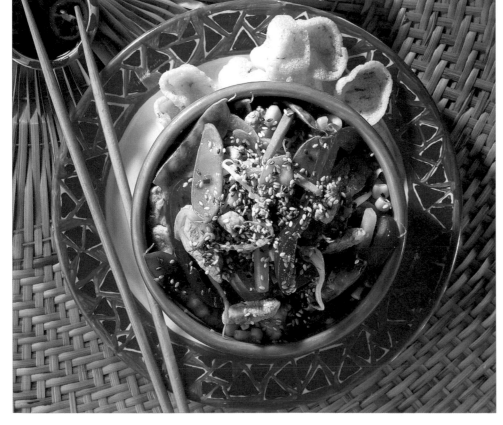

| — NUTRITION NOTES — | |
| --- | --- |
| Per portion: | |
| Energy | 327kcals |
| Protein | 24.95g |
| Fat | 7.90g |
| Saturated fat | 1.89g |
| Carbohydrate | 40.81g |
| Fiber | 4.77g |
| Added sugar | 5.38g |
| Sodium | 0.73g |

# Lamb with Vegetables

A good variety of vegetables makes this a healthy dish.

## INGREDIENTS

*Serves 6*
juice of 1 lemon
1 tablespoon soy sauce
1 tablespoon dry sherry
1 garlic clove, crushed
2 teaspoons chopped fresh rosemary
6 lean lamb chops
1 red onion, cut into 8 pieces
1 onion, cut into 8 pieces
1 red, 1 yellow and 1 green bell pepper,
   seeded and cut into chunks
4 zucchini, thickly sliced
4½ cups button mushrooms
2 tablespoons olive oil
4 plum tomatoes, peeled
14-ounce can baby corn
4 tablespoons chopped fresh basil
1–2 tablespoons balsamic vinegar
salt and ground black pepper
basil sprigs, to garnish
baked potatoes, to serve

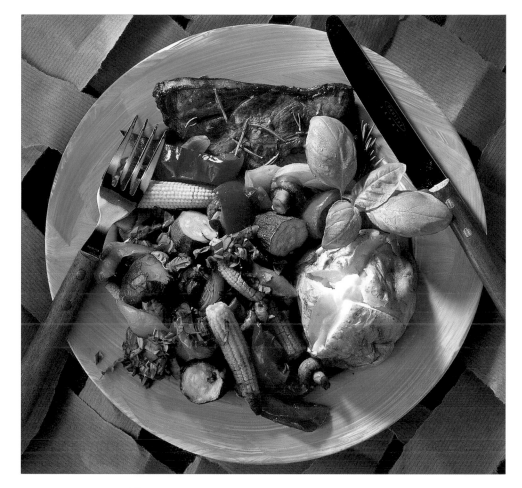

*1* In a shallow dish, mix together the lemon juice, soy sauce, sherry, garlic and rosemary. Coat the lamb chops in the marinade. Cover and refrigerate for 2 hours.

*2* Preheat the oven to 400°F. Put the onions, peppers, zucchini and mushrooms in a roasting pan, drizzle with the oil and toss. Bake for 25 minutes.

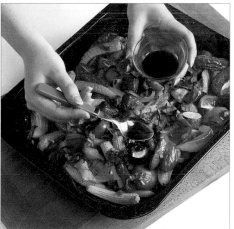

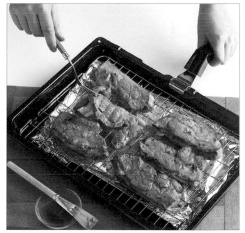

*3* Quarter the tomatoes and stir in with the corn. Bake for another 10 minutes, until all the vegetables are just tender and slightly browned at the edges. Then add the chopped fresh basil, sprinkle with the balsamic vinegar, and season to taste, stirring thoroughly to mix well.

*4* Preheat the broiler. Place the lamb chops under medium heat for about 6 minutes on each side, until cooked, turning over once. Brush the chops with any remaining marinade while they are cooking, to prevent them from drying out. Place the chops on individual serving plates with the vegetables, garnish with basil sprigs and serve with potatoes.

| NUTRITION NOTES | |
| --- | --- |
| Per portion: | |
| Energy | 273kcals |
| Protein | 26.95g |
| Fat | 12.60g |
| Saturated fat | 4.22g |
| Carbohydrate | 13.15g |
| Fiber | 4.99g |
| Added sugar | 0.10g |
| Sodium | 0.91g |

# Spiced Lamb and Vegetable Couscous

A delicious stew of tender lamb and vegetables, served with plenty of couscous.

### INGREDIENTS

*Serves 6*

12 ounces lean lamb fillet, cut
   into ¾-inch cubes
2 tablespoons whole-wheat
   flour, seasoned
2 teaspoons sunflower oil
1 onion, chopped
2 garlic cloves, crushed
1 red bell pepper, seeded and diced
1 teaspoon ground coriander
1 teaspoon ground cumin
1 teaspoon ground allspice
½ teaspoon hot chili powder
1¼ cups lamb stock
14-ounce can chopped tomatoes
8 ounces carrots, sliced
6 ounces parsnips, sliced
6 ounces zucchini, sliced
2½ cups closed cap
   mushrooms, quartered
8 ounces frozen fava or lima beans
¾ cup golden raisins
2¾ cups quick-cook couscous
salt and ground black pepper
fresh cilantro, to garnish

---

#### — NUTRITION NOTES —

Per portion:
| | |
|---|---|
| Energy | 439kcals |
| Protein | 23.29g |
| Fat | 8.15g |
| Saturated fat | 2.57g |
| Carbohydrate | 72.98g |
| Fiber | 7.34g |
| Added sugar | 0.00g |
| Sodium | 0.18g |

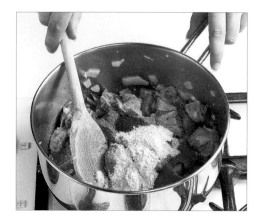

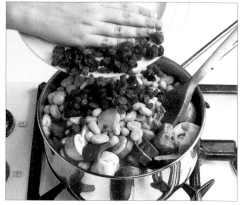

*2* Add any remaining flour and the spices and cook for 1 minute, stirring continuously.

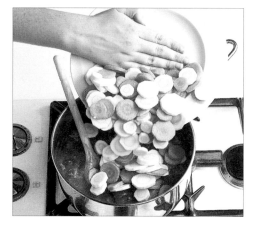

*3* Gradually add the stock, continuing to stir, then add the tomatoes, carrots and parsnips, and mix well.

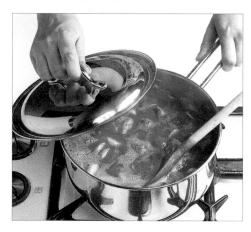

*4* Bring to a boil, stirring, then cover and simmer for 30 minutes, stirring occasionally.

*1* Toss the lamb fillet in the seasoned flour. Heat the oil in a large saucepan and add the lamb, onion, garlic and pepper. Cook for 5 minutes, stirring frequently.

*5* Add the zucchini, mushrooms, beans and raisins. Cover, return to a boil and simmer, stirring occasionally, for another 20–30 minutes, until the lamb and vegetables are tender. Season to taste.

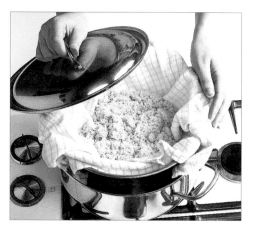

*6* Meanwhile, soak the couscous and steam in a colander lined with a dish towel over a pan of boiling water for 20 minutes, until cooked or according to the package instructions. Pile the cooked couscous onto a warmed serving platter or individual plates, and top with the lamb and vegetable stew. Garnish with fresh cilantro and serve immediately.

---

#### — VARIATION —

As a tasty alternative to couscous, you might prefer to serve this lamb and vegetable stew on a bed of cooked bulgur wheat or brown rice.

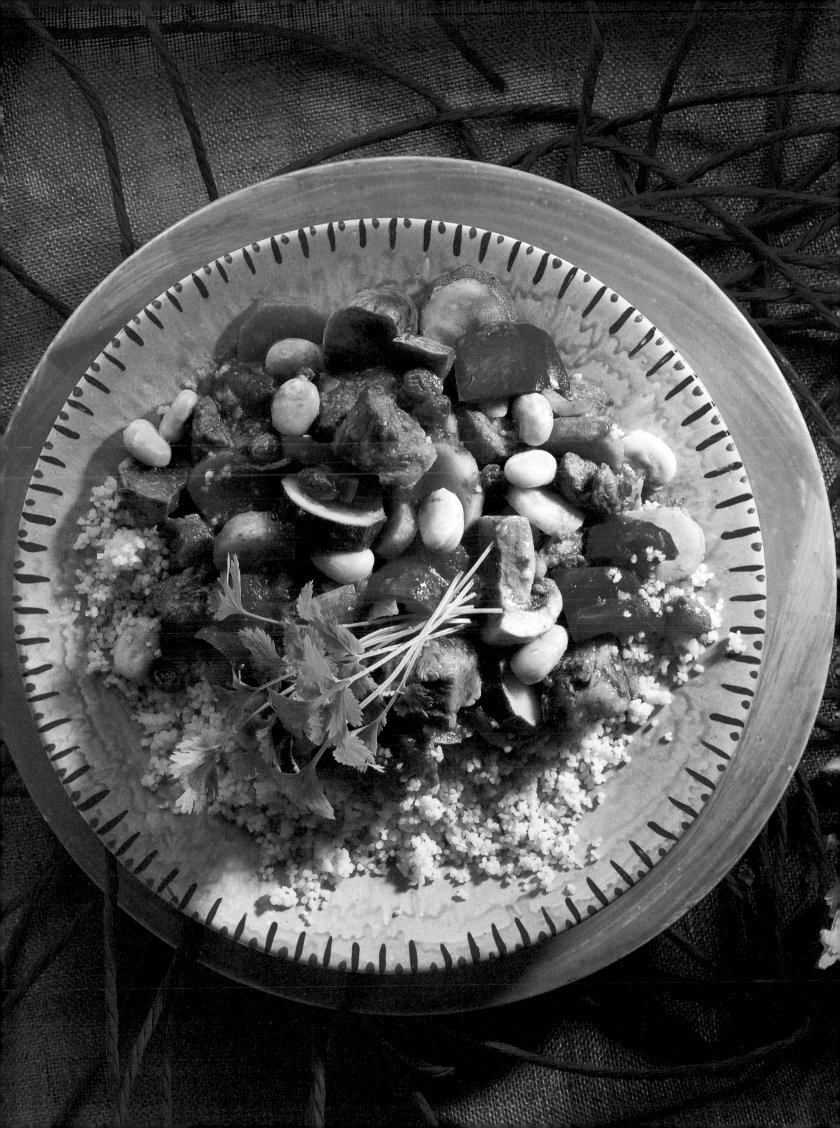

# Chicken and Bean Risotto

Brown rice, red kidney beans, corn and broccoli all add extra fiber to this risotto.

### INGREDIENTS

*Serves 4–6*

1 onion, chopped
2 garlic cloves, crushed
1 fresh red chile, seeded and
 finely chopped
2¼ cups mushrooms, sliced
2 celery stalks, chopped
1 cup long-grain brown rice
scant 2 cups stock
⅔ cup white wine
14-ounce can red kidney beans
8 ounces skinless, boneless chicken
 breast, diced
7-ounce can corn kernels
¼ cup golden raisins
6 ounces small broccoli florets
2–3 tablespoons chopped fresh
 mixed herbs
salt and ground black pepper

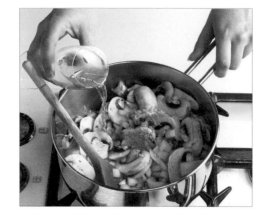

*1* Put the onion, garlic, chile, mushrooms, celery, rice, stock and wine in a saucepan. Cover, bring to a boil and simmer for 15 minutes.

--- COOK'S TIP ---

When preparing fresh chiles, wear gloves to protect your hands or wash your hands well afterward and avoid touching your eyes. Use 1 teaspoon hot chili powder in place of the fresh chile, if you like.

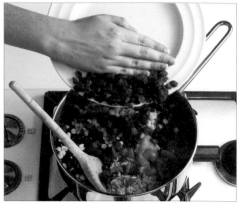

*2* Rinse and drain the kidney beans. Stir the chicken, kidney beans, corn and raisins into the pan. Cook for another 20 minutes, until almost all the liquid has been absorbed.

*3* Cook the broccoli in boiling water for 5 minutes, then drain.

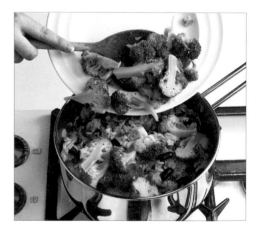

*4* Stir the broccoli and chopped herbs into the risotto, season to taste and serve immediately.

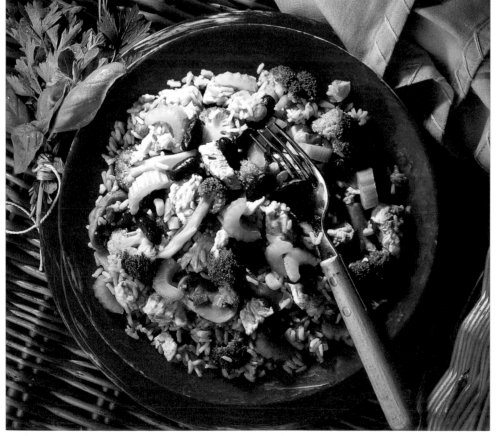

--- NUTRITION NOTES ---

| Per portion: | |
| --- | --- |
| Energy | 563kcals |
| Protein | 31.01g |
| Fat | 5.73g |
| Saturated fat | 1.31g |
| Carbohydrate | 96.85g |
| Fiber | 8.72g |
| Added sugar | 0.02g |
| Sodium | 0.66g |

# Smoked Bacon and Green Bean Pasta Salad

A tasty pasta salad subtly flavored with smoked bacon and tossed together in a light, flavorful dressing.

## INGREDIENTS

*Serves 4*

3 cups whole-wheat pasta twists
1½ cups green beans
8 strips lean smoked Canadian
 bacon, rind and fat removed
12 ounces cherry tomatoes, halved
2 bunches scallions, chopped
14-ounce can chickpeas, rinsed
 and drained
6 tablespoons tomato juice
2 tablespoons balsamic vinegar
1 teaspoon ground cumin
1 teaspoon ground coriander
2 tablespoons chopped
 fresh cilantro
salt and ground black pepper

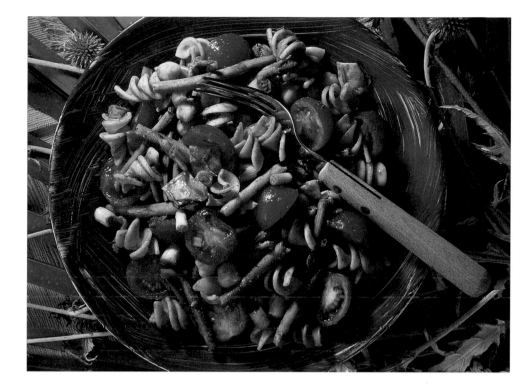

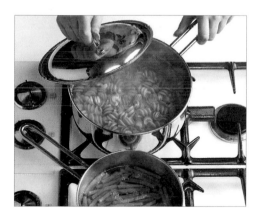

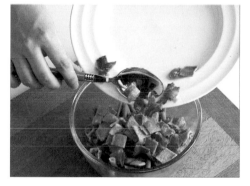

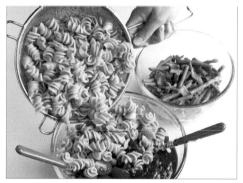

*1* Cook the pasta in a large saucepan of lightly salted, boiling water for 10–12 minutes, until al dente. Meanwhile, trim and halve the green beans and cook them in boiling water for about 5 minutes, until tender. Drain thoroughly and keep warm.

*2* Preheat the broiler and cook the bacon for 2–3 minutes on each side, until cooked. Dice the bacon and add to the beans.

*3* Put the tomatoes, scallions and chickpeas in a bowl, and mix together. In a small bowl, mix together the tomato juice, vinegar, spices, fresh cilantro and seasoning, and pour this over the tomato mixture.

*4* Drain the pasta thoroughly, and add to the tomato mixture with the beans and bacon. Toss all the ingredients together to mix, and serve warm or cold.

---

### COOK'S TIP

Always thoroughly rinse any canned pulses that you use before adding them to the dish, in order to remove as much of the brine (salt water) as possible.

---

### NUTRITION NOTES

| Per portion: | |
| --- | --- |
| Energy | 444kcals |
| Protein | 28.43g |
| Fat | 8.67g |
| Saturated fat | 1.98g |
| Carbohydrate | 68.69g |
| Fiber | 13.43g |
| Added sugar | 0.00g |
| Sodium | 1.26g |

# Bean and Ham Lasagne

Serve this scrumptious lasagne with a light and wholesome salad and fresh bread.

## INGREDIENTS

*Serves 6*

2 teaspoons olive oil
3 cups leeks, sliced
1 garlic clove, crushed
3 cups mushrooms, sliced
2 zucchini, sliced
12 ounces baby fava beans
2 cups lean smoked ham, diced
5 tablespoons chopped fresh parsley
2 tablespoons chopped fresh chives
4 tablespoons half-fat spread
½ cup whole-wheat flour
2½ cups skim milk
1¼ cups vegetable stock, cooled
6 ounces low-fat cheese
1 teaspoon smooth mustard
8 ounces whole-wheat lasagne
½ cup fresh whole-wheat bread crumbs
1 tablespoon grated Parmesan cheese
salt and ground black pepper
fresh herb sprigs, to garnish

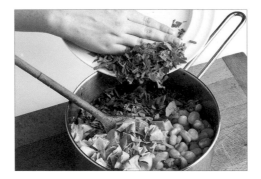

*2* Remove the pan from heat, and stir in the fava beans, ham and herbs. Set aside.

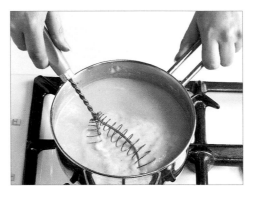

*3* Make the cheese sauce. Put the half-fat spread, flour, milk and stock in a heavy-bottomed saucepan and heat gently, whisking continuously, until the sauce comes to a boil and thickens. Simmer gently for 3 minutes, stirring. Grate the cheese.

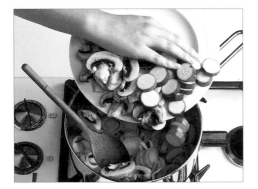

*1* Preheat the oven to 350°F. Heat the oil in a saucepan, add the leeks and garlic and cook for 3 minutes, stirring constantly, until softened. Add the mushrooms and zucchini and cook for 5 minutes, stirring occasionally.

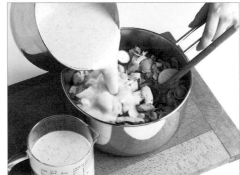

*4* Remove the pan from heat, add the mustard and grated cheese and stir until the cheese has melted and is well blended. Season to taste. Reserve scant 2 cups of cheese sauce and set aside. Mix the remaining sauce with the ham and vegetables.

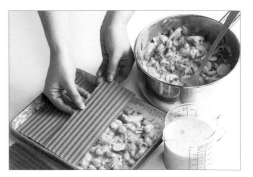

*5* Spoon half the ham mixture over the base of a shallow ovenproof dish or baking pan. Cover this with half the pasta. Repeat these layers with the remaining ham mixture and pasta, then pour the reserved cheese sauce over the pasta to cover it completely.

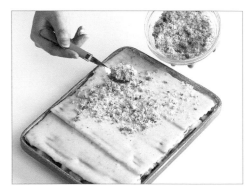

*6* Mix together the fresh whole-wheat bread crumbs and the grated Parmesan cheese, and sprinkle this mixture over the lasagne. Bake for 45–60 minutes, until the lasagne is cooked and golden brown on top. Garnish with fresh herb sprigs and serve immediately.

| — NUTRITION NOTES — | |
| --- | --- |
| Per portion: | |
| Energy | 448kcals |
| Protein | 38.45g |
| Fat | 13.05g |
| Saturated fat | 5.07g |
| Carbohydrate | 46.16g |
| Fiber | 10.86g |
| Added sugar | 0.02g |
| Sodium | 0.50g |

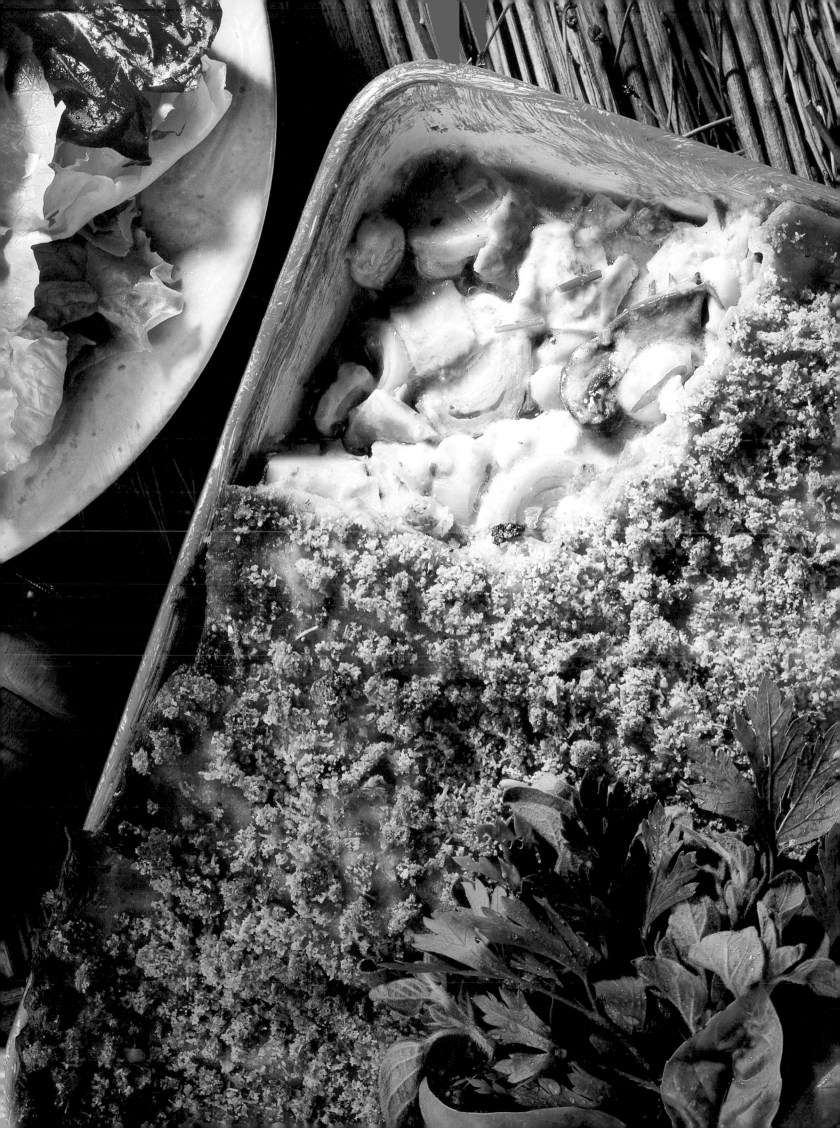

# Chicken and Bean Casserole

A delicious combination of chicken, tarragon and mixed beans with a potato topping.

## Ingredients

*Serves 6*

2 pounds potatoes
½ cup reduced-fat aged
  Cheddar cheese, finely grated
2½ cups plus 2–3 tablespoons skim milk
2 tablespoons chopped fresh chives
2 leeks, sliced
1 onion, sliced
2 tablespoons dry white wine
3 tablespoons half-fat spread
⅓ cup whole-wheat flour
1¼ cups chicken stock, cooled
12 ounces cooked skinless, boneless
  chicken breast, diced
3 cups cremini mushrooms, sliced
11-ounce can red kidney beans
14-ounce can flageolet beans
14-ounce can black-eyed beans
2–3 tablespoons chopped
  fresh tarragon
salt and ground black pepper

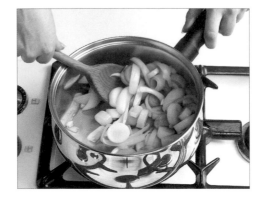

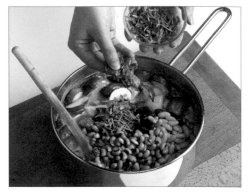

2 Meanwhile, put the leeks and onion in a saucepan with the wine. Cover, and cook gently for 10 minutes, until the vegetables are just tender, stirring occasionally.

5 Rinse and drain all the beans, and add to the sauce. Stir in the tarragon and seasoning to taste. Heat, stirring gently, until the chicken mixture is piping hot.

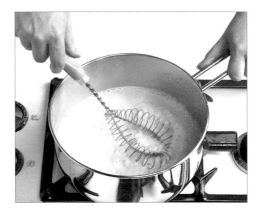

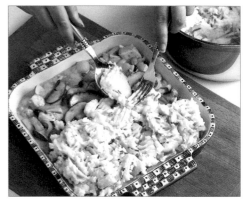

3 In the meantime, put the half-fat spread, flour, remaining milk and stock in a saucepan. Heat gently, whisking continuously, until the sauce comes to a boil and thickens. Simmer gently for 3 minutes, stirring.

4 Remove the pan from heat and add the leek mixture, chicken and mushrooms, and mix well.

6 Transfer the hot chicken and bean mixture to an ovenproof dish. Then spoon or pipe the mashed potato over the top so that it covers the filling completely. Put the dish in the oven and bake for about 30 minutes, until the potato topping is crisp and golden brown. Serve immediately.

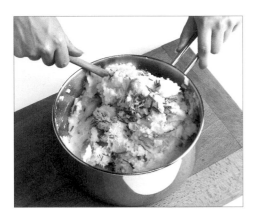

1 Preheat the oven to 400°F. Cut the potatoes into chunks and cook in lightly salted boiling water for 15–20 minutes, until tender. Drain and mash. Add the cheese, 2–3 tablespoons milk and chives, season to taste, and mix well. Keep warm and set aside.

--- Variation ---

Sweet potatoes in place of standard potatoes work just as well in this recipe, and turkey or lean ham can be used instead of the chicken for a change.

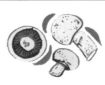

--- Nutrition Notes ---

Per portion:

| | |
|---|---|
| Energy | 541kcals |
| Protein | 44.98g |
| Fat | 9.36g |
| Saturated fat | 2.85g |
| Carbohydrate | 72.49g |
| Fiber | 16.46g |
| Added sugar | 0.01g |
| Sodium | 0.62g |

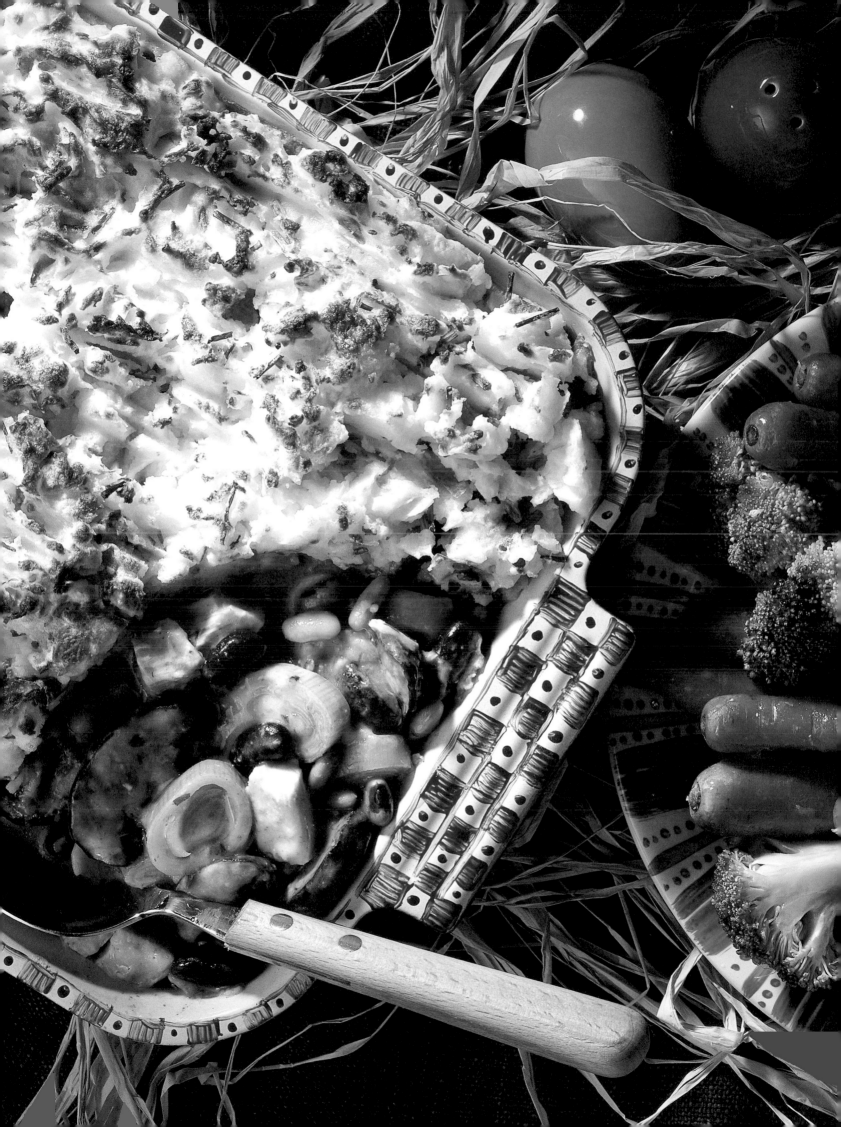

# Country Chicken Casserole

Succulent chicken pieces are cooked in a rich vegetable sauce and are particularly good served with brown rice.

## INGREDIENTS

*Serves 4*
2 chicken breasts, skinned
2 chicken legs, skinned
2 tablespoons whole-wheat flour
1 tablespoon sunflower oil
1¼ cups chicken stock
1¼ cups white wine
2 tablespoons passata (sieved tomatoes)
1 tablespoon tomato paste
4 strips lean smoked Canadian bacon
1 large onion, sliced
1 garlic clove, crushed
1 green bell pepper, seeded and sliced
3 cups button mushrooms
8 ounces carrots, sliced
1 bouquet garni
8 ounces frozen Brussels sprouts
1½ cups frozen tiny peas
salt and ground black pepper
chopped fresh parsley, to garnish
brown rice, to serve

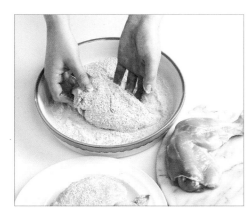

*1* Preheat the oven to 350°F. Coat the chicken pieces with seasoned flour.

--- VARIATION ---

Use fresh Brussels sprouts and peas if they are available, and use red wine in place of white for a change.

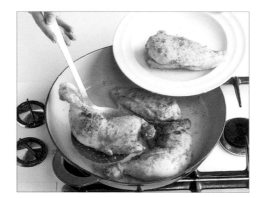

*2* Heat the oil in a large, flameproof casserole, add the chicken and cook until browned. Remove the chicken, using a slotted spoon, and set aside.

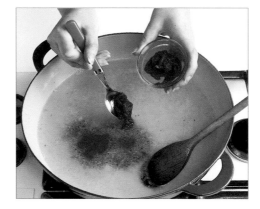

*3* Add the remaining flour to the pan and cook for 1 minute. Gradually stir in the stock and wine, then add the passata and tomato paste.

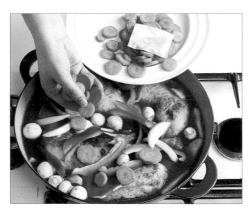

*4* Bring to a boil, stirring continuously, then add the chicken, bacon, onion, garlic, green pepper, mushrooms, carrots and bouquet garni and stir. Cover and bake for 1½ hours, stirring once or twice.

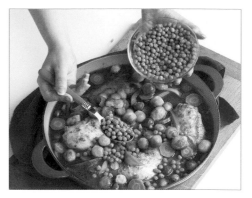

*5* Stir in the Brussels sprouts and peas, re-cover and bake for another 30 minutes.

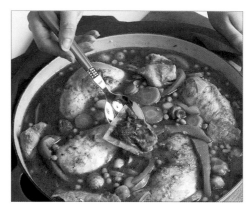

*6* Remove and discard the bouquet garni. Add seasoning to the casserole, garnish with the chopped fresh parsley and serve with brown rice.

--- NUTRITION NOTES ---

Per portion:
| | |
|---|---|
| Energy | 360kcals |
| Protein | 37.83g |
| Fat | 9.00g |
| Saturated fat | 2.11g |
| Carbohydrate | 21.55g |
| Fiber | 8.51g |
| Added sugar | 0.01g |
| Sodium | 0.71g |

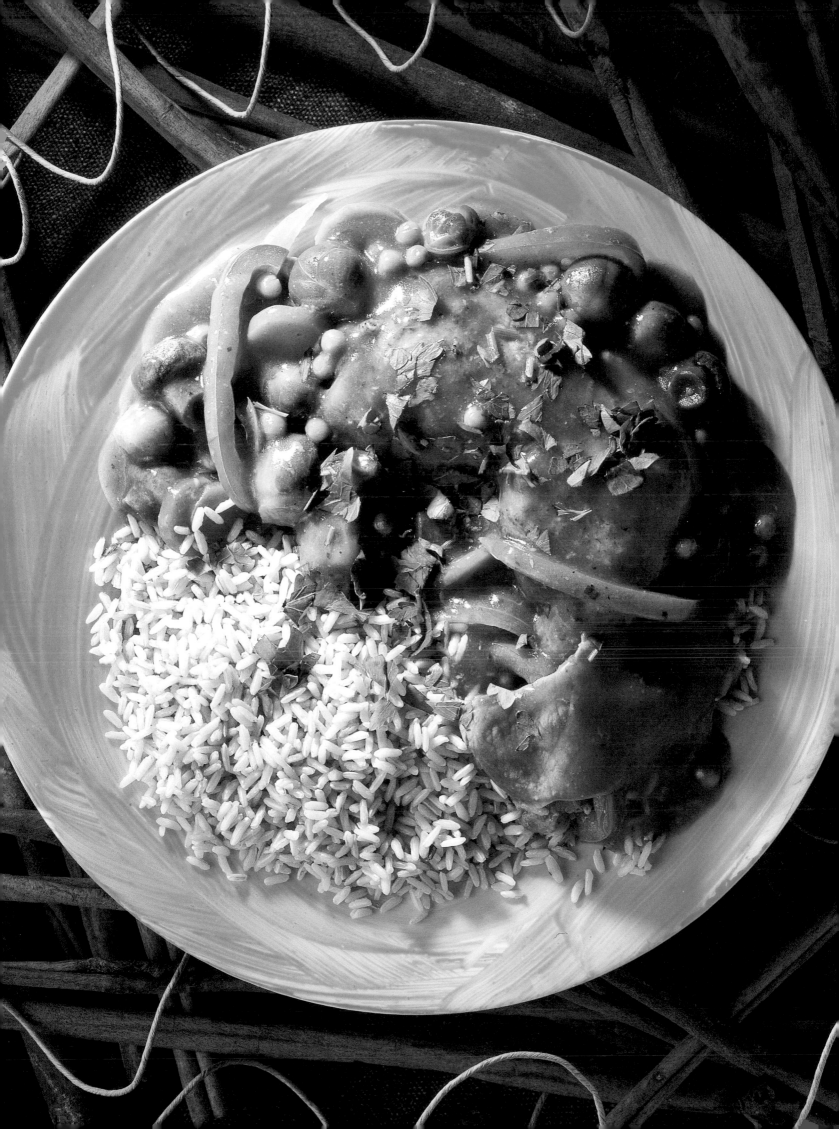

# Salmon and Broccoli Pilaf

This pilaf is an excellent choice for an informal supper.

## Ingredients

*Serves 4*

1 red onion, chopped
1 garlic clove, crushed
4 celery stalks, chopped
1 yellow bell pepper, seeded and diced
1 cup brown basmati rice
2½ cups fish stock
1¼ cups white wine
14-ounce can pink salmon, drained and flaked
14-ounce can red kidney beans, rinsed and drained
12 ounces small broccoli florets
3 tablespoons chopped fresh parsley
1–2 tablespoons light soy sauce
salt and ground black pepper
1 ounce toasted sliced almonds, to garnish

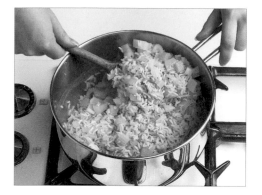

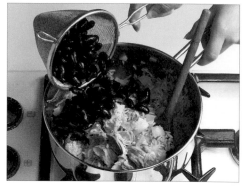

*1* Put the onion, garlic, celery, pepper, rice, stock and wine in a saucepan and bring to a boil, stirring. Simmer, uncovered, for 25–30 minutes, until almost all the liquid has been absorbed, stirring occasionally.

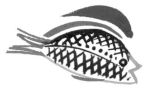

*2* Stir the salmon and kidney beans into the rice mixture. Cook gently for another 5–10 minutes, until the pilaf is piping hot.

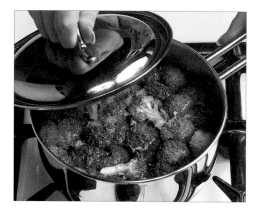

*3* Meanwhile, cook the broccoli florets in boiling water for about 5 minutes, until tender. Drain thoroughly and keep warm.

*4* Fold the broccoli gently into the pilaf, then stir in the parsley and soy sauce, and season to taste. Garnish with toasted sliced almonds, and serve immediately.

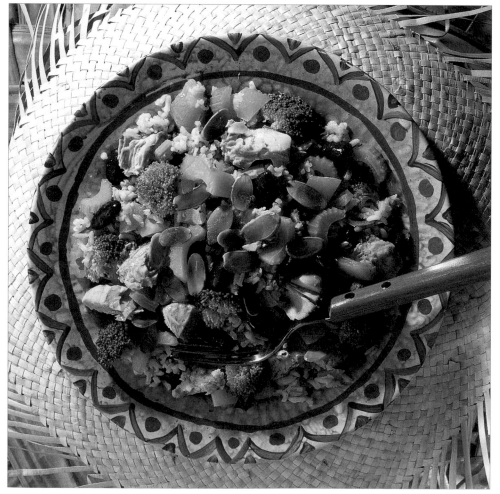

### Nutrition Notes

Per portion:

| | |
|---|---|
| Energy | 550kcals |
| Protein | 33.38g |
| Fat | 11.98g |
| Saturated fat | 2.00g |
| Carbohydrate | 69.55g |
| Fiber | 9.51g |
| Added sugar | 0.34g |
| Sodium | 1.39g |

# Oatmeal-crusted Mackerel

An appetizing way of serving fresh mackerel. Accompany with baked potatoes and cooked snow peas for a tasty and filling meal.

## INGREDIENTS

*Serves 4*
4 mackerel, each weighing about
    6–8 ounces
juice of 1 lemon
½ cup fine oatmeal
½ cup medium oatmeal
2 tablespoons chopped fresh
    mixed herbs
salt and ground black pepper
tomato quarters and fresh herb
    sprigs, to garnish
baked potatoes and snow peas, to serve

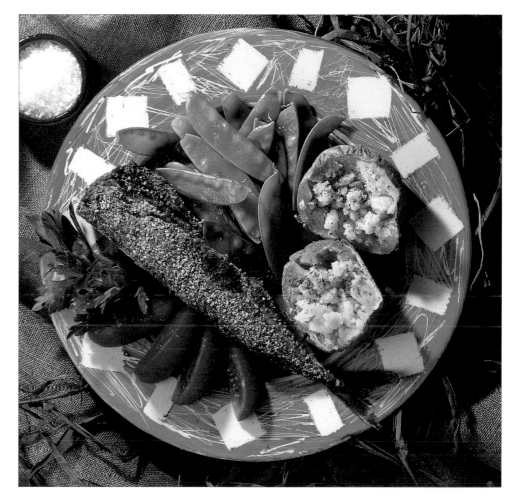

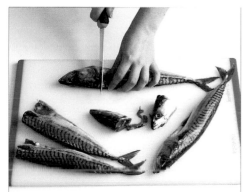

*1* Remove and discard the heads from the mackerel, then clean the fish thoroughly.

*2* Sprinkle the inside of each mackerel with lemon juice and season according to taste.

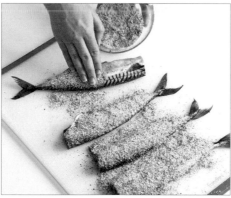

*3* Mix together the two oatmeals and herbs, and press the mixture firmly onto the outside of each fish.

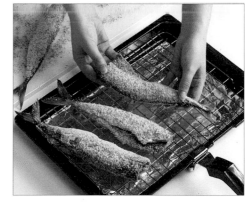

*4* Preheat the broiler. Broil the fish under fairly high heat for 6–8 minutes, turning once, until it is tender and is just beginning to flake. Garnish with tomato quarters and fresh herb sprigs, and serve with baked potatoes and snow peas.

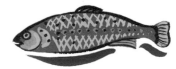

---

### NUTRITION NOTES

Per portion:

| | |
|---|---|
| Energy | 480kcals |
| Protein | 36.30g |
| Fat | 30.15g |
| Saturated fat | 6.18g |
| Carbohydrate | 16.63g |
| Fiber | 1.88g |
| Added sugar | 0.00g |
| Sodium | 0.10g |

---

### VARIATION

Fresh sardines or trout can be used in place of the mackerel in this recipe and are equally tasty.

# Tuna, Chickpea and Cherry Tomato Salad

This healthy salad is easy to prepare and makes a light, satisfying meal when served with whole-wheat bread. Only a little oil is used for the dressing, but it is very flavorful.

## INGREDIENTS

*Serves 6*

1 teaspoon olive oil
1 garlic clove, crushed
1 teaspoon ground coriander
1 teaspoon garam masala
1 teaspoon hot chili powder
½ cup tomato juice
2 tablespoons balsamic vinegar
dash of Tabasco sauce
1½ pounds cherry tomatoes, halved
½ cucumber, sliced
1 bunch radishes, sliced
1 bunch scallions, chopped
2 ounces watercress
2 14-ounce cans chickpeas,
  rinsed and drained
14-ounce can tuna in brine,
  drained and flaked
1 tablespoon chopped fresh parsley
1 tablespoon chopped fresh chives
salt and ground black pepper

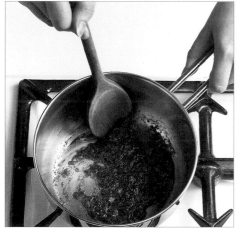

*1* Heat the oil in a small saucepan. Add the garlic and spices, and cook gently for 1 minute, stirring.

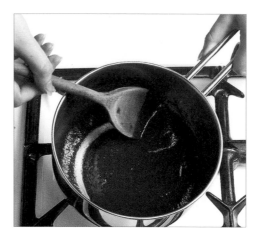

*2* Stir in the tomato juice, vinegar and Tabasco sauce, and heat gently until the mixture is boiling. Remove the pan from heat, and set aside to cool slightly.

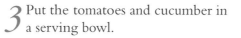

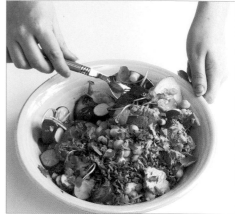

*3* Put the tomatoes and cucumber in a serving bowl.

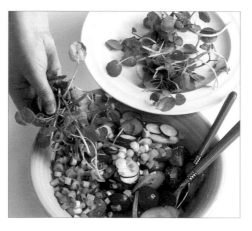

*4* Add the prepared radishes, scallions and watercress to the tomato mixture.

*5* Gently stir in the chickpeas, the tuna and the herbs.

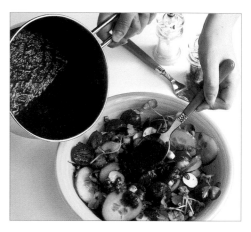

*6* Pour the tomato dressing over the salad and toss the ingredients together to mix. Season and serve.

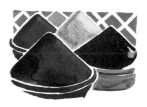

| NUTRITION NOTES | |
| --- | --- |
| Per portion: | |
| Energy | 198kcals |
| Protein | 20.98g |
| Fat | 4.30g |
| Saturated Fat | 0.62g |
| Carbohydrate | 20.70g |
| Fiber | 5.88g |
| Added Sugar | 0.00g |
| Sodium | 0.45g |

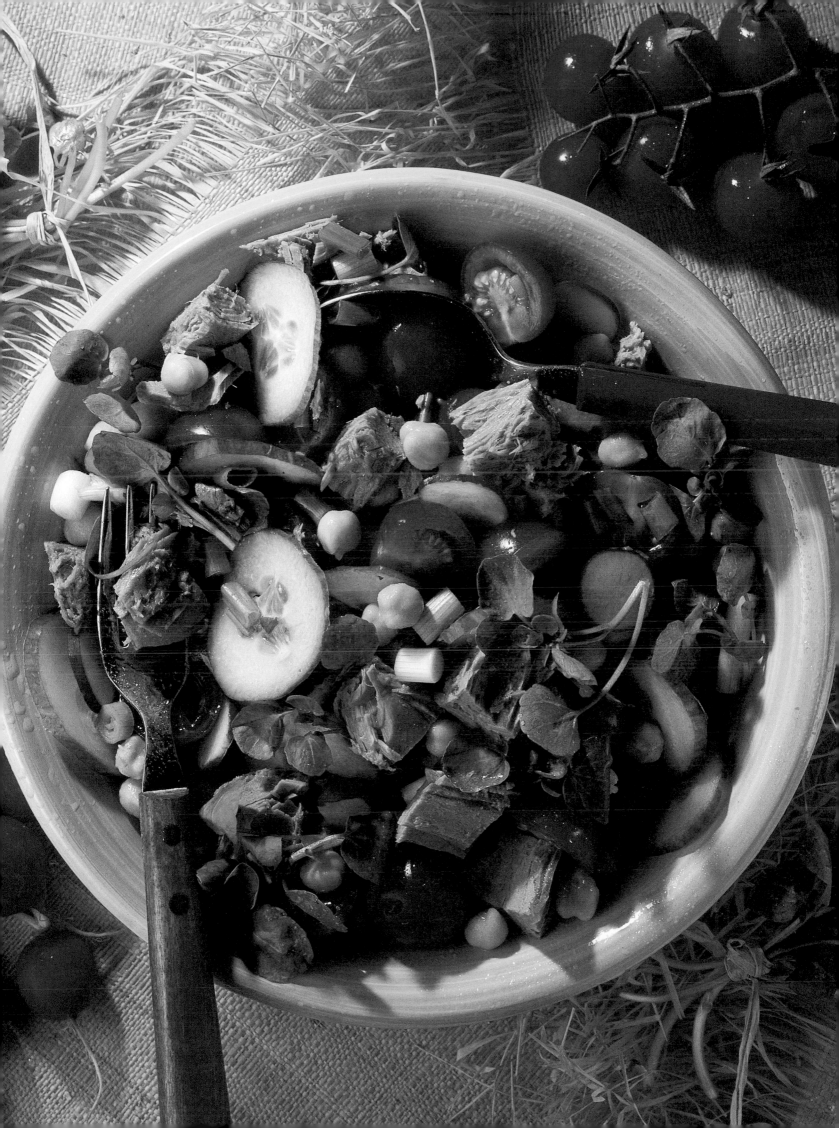

# Spicy Seafood and Okra Stew

This spicy seafood dish is good accompanied by herbed brown rice. Heat the seafood mixture until piping hot before serving.

## INGREDIENTS

*Serves 4–6*

2 teaspoons olive oil
1 onion, chopped
1 garlic clove, crushed
2 celery stalks, chopped
1 red bell pepper, seeded and diced
1 teaspoon each ground coriander, ground cumin and ground ginger
½ teaspoon hot chili powder
½ teaspoon garam masala
2 tablespoons whole-wheat flour
1¼ cups each fish stock and dry white wine
8-ounce can chopped tomatoes
8 ounces okra, trimmed and sliced
3 cups mushrooms, sliced
1 pound frozen cooked, shelled seafood, defrosted
1 cup frozen corn kernels
1 cup long-grain brown rice
2–3 tablespoons chopped fresh mixed herbs
salt and ground black pepper
flat-leaf parsley sprigs, to garnish

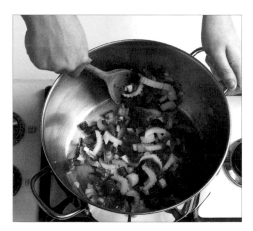

*1* Heat the oil in a large saucepan. Add the onion, garlic, celery and red pepper and cook for 5 minutes, stirring occasionally.

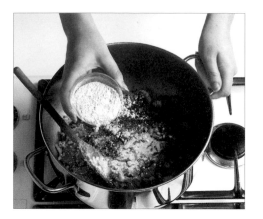

*2* Add the spices and cook for 1 minute, stirring, then add the flour and cook for 1 minute more, continuing to stir.

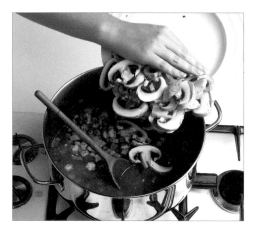

*3* Gradually stir in the stock and wine, and add the tomatoes, okra and mushrooms. Bring to a boil, stirring continuously, then cover and simmer for 20 minutes, stirring

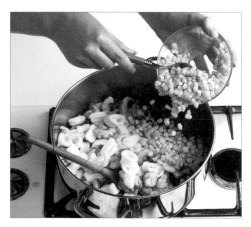

*4* Stir in the seafood and corn. Cook for 10–15 minutes, until hot.

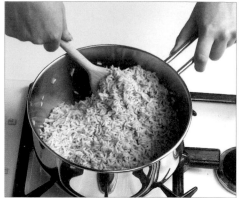

*5* Meanwhile, cook the brown rice in a large saucepan of lightly salted boiling water for about 35 minutes, until just tender.

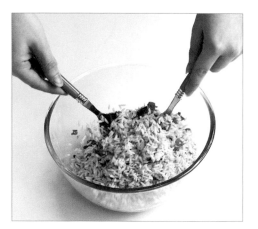

*6* Rinse the cooked rice in fresh boiling water, and drain thoroughly. Then toss the rice together with the mixed herbs to mix well. Finally, season the stew, and serve on a bed of the herbed rice. Garnish with flat-leaf parsley sprigs.

| — NUTRITION NOTES — | |
|---|---|
| Per portion: | |
| Energy | 541kcals |
| Protein | 34.96g |
| Fat | 7.18g |
| Saturated fat | 1.42g |
| Carbohydrate | 76.05g |
| Fiber | 7.25g |
| Added sugar | 0.01g |
| Sodium | 1.35g |

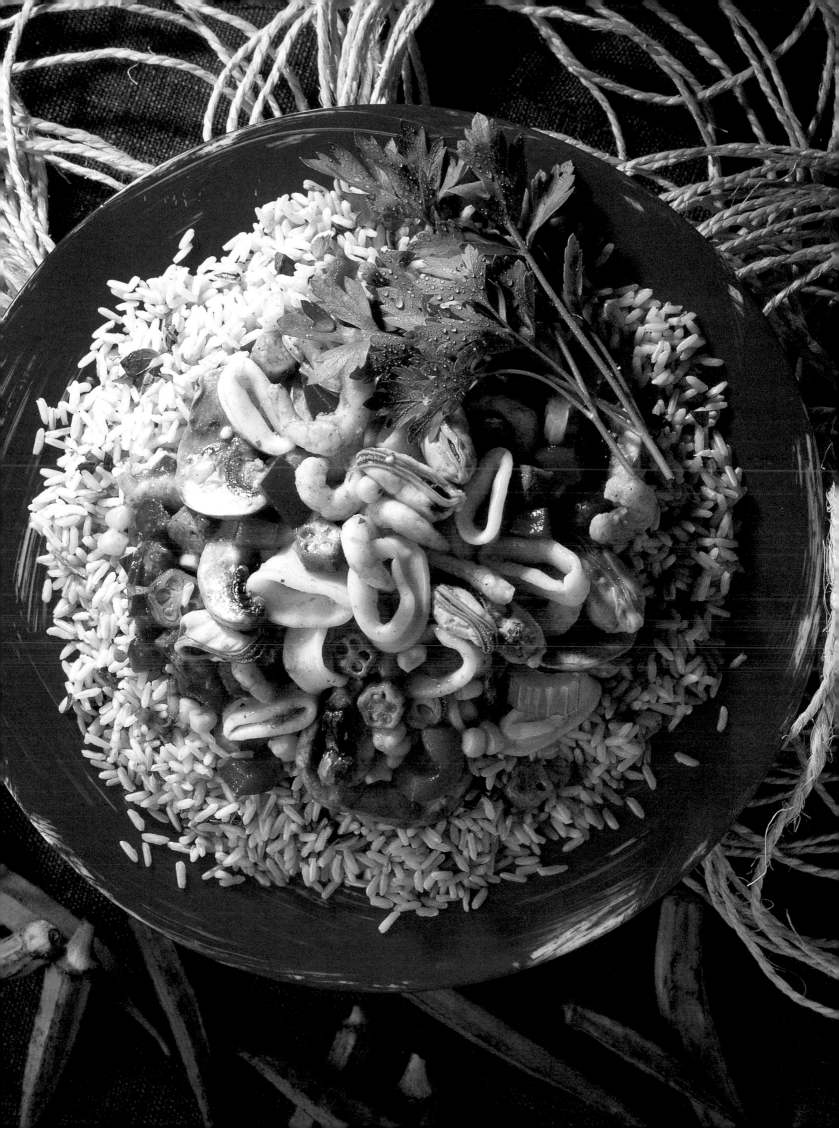

# Salmon, Zucchini and Corn Frittata

Serve this unusual frittata as a delicious and exciting change from an omelet, with a mixed tomato and bell pepper salad and warm whole-wheat bread rolls.

## INGREDIENTS

*Serves 4–6*
2 teaspoons olive oil
1 onion, chopped
1⅓ cups thinly sliced zucchini
8 ounces boiled potatoes (with skins left on), diced
3 eggs, plus 2 egg whites
2 tablespoons skim milk
7-ounce can pink salmon in brine, drained and flaked
7-ounce can corn kernels, drained
2 teaspoons dried mixed herbs
½ cup reduced-fat aged Cheddar cheese, finely grated
salt and ground black pepper
chopped fresh mixed herbs and basil leaves, to garnish
pepper and tomato salad, to serve

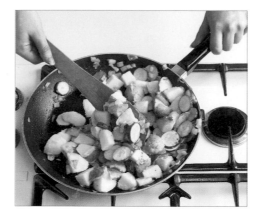

*2* Add the potatoes and cook for 5 minutes, stirring occasionally.

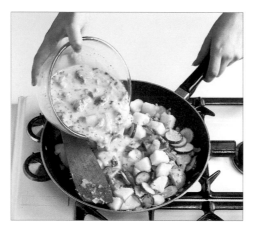

*3* Beat the eggs, egg whites and milk together, add the salmon, corn, dried herbs and seasoning to taste and pour the mixture evenly over the vegetables.

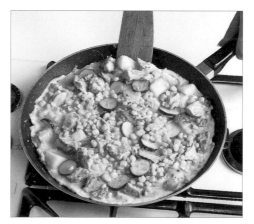

*4* Cook over medium heat until the eggs are beginning to set and the frittata has begun to turn golden brown underneath.

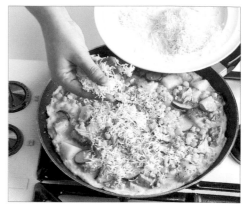

*5* Preheat the broiler. Sprinkle the cheese over the frittata, and place it under medium heat, until the cheese has melted and the top is golden brown.

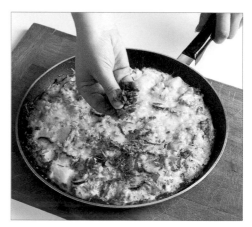

*6* Sprinkle the cooked frittata with plenty of chopped fresh herbs, and garnish with basil leaves. Serve the frittata immediately, while hot, cut into wedges and accompanied by a pepper and tomato salad.

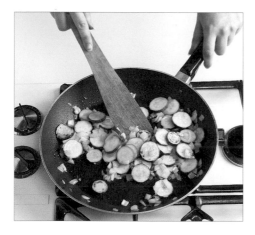

*1* Heat the oil in a large, nonstick frying pan. Add the onion and zucchini, and cook for 5 minutes, stirring occasionally.

---

VARIATION

Use canned tuna or crab in place of the salmon, if you like.

---

— NUTRITION NOTES —

Per portion:
| | |
|---|---|
| Energy | 336kcals |
| Protein | 25.85g |
| Fat | 12.20g |
| Saturated fat | 3.57g |
| Carbohydrate | 32.83g |
| Fiber | 4.34g |
| Added sugar | 0.00g |
| Sodium | 0.49g |

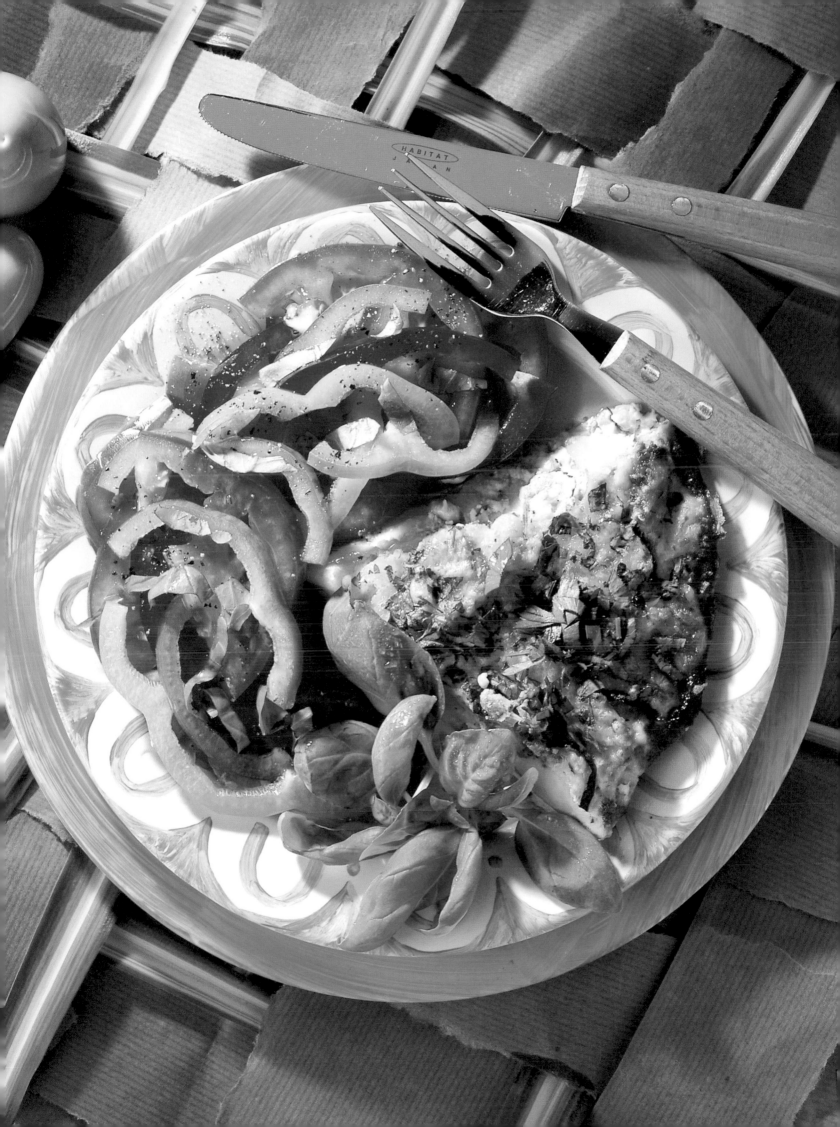

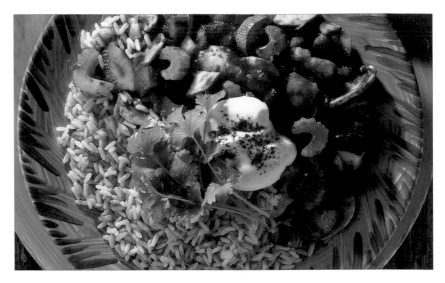

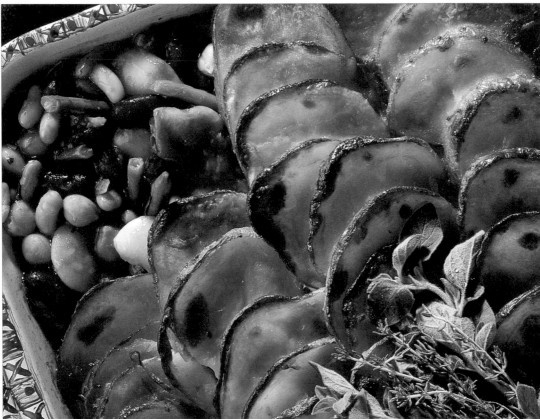

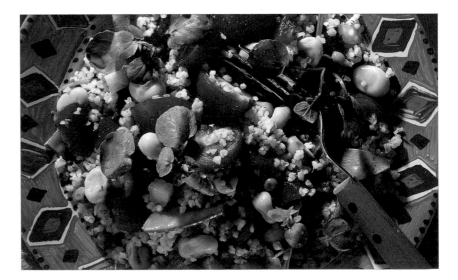

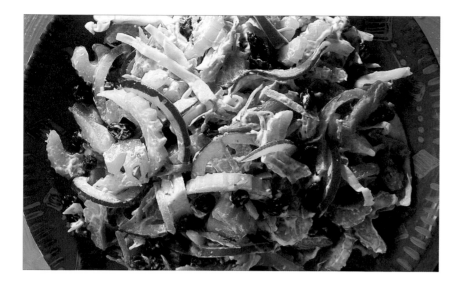

# VEGETARIAN DISHES

Vegetarians have a head start on the rest of us when it comes to fiber in the diet, since they already value vegetables, pulses, pasta, rice, nuts and seed, and consume plenty of whole foods. Most vegetarians naturally eat a healthy, well-balanced diet. However, there are still some who take the less healthful option, choosing processed foods like white rice or pasta drenched in cream sauce and topped with cheese. For them, this chapter offers fabulous fiber-rich alternatives, such as Vegetable Paella or Zucchini, Corn and Plum Tomato Pizza. Recipes like Sweet-and-Sour Mixed Bean Hot Pot and Vegetable Chili prove that a vegetarian meal can be just as substantial and filling as one using meat. Whatever your preference, though, these delicious dishes are all guaranteed to go down well!

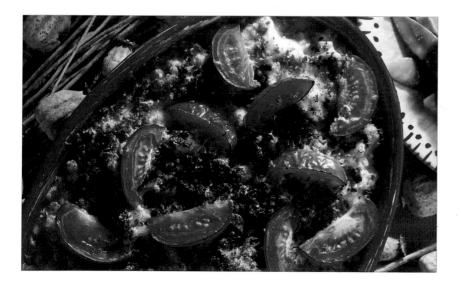

# Vegetable Paella

This recipe makes a delicious change from the traditional, seafood-based paella.

### INGREDIENTS

*Serves 6*
1 onion, chopped
2 garlic cloves, crushed
2 cups sliced leeks
3 celery stalks, chopped
1 red bell pepper, seeded and sliced
2 zucchini, sliced
2¼ cups cremini
  mushrooms, sliced
14-ounce can cannellini beans
1½ cups frozen peas
2¼ cups long-grain brown rice
3¾ cups vegetable stock
¼ cup dry white wine
a few saffron strands
8 ounces cherry tomatoes, halved
3–4 tablespoons fresh mixed herbs
salt and ground black pepper
celery leaves and cherry tomatoes,
  to garnish
lemon wedges, to serve

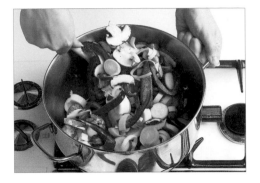

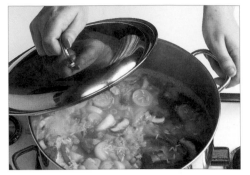

1 Put the onion, garlic, leeks, celery, pepper, zucchini and mushrooms in a large saucepan, and mix together.

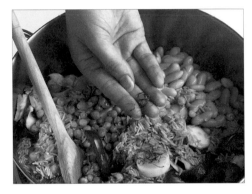

2 Rinse and drain the cannellini beans. Add them to the pan with the peas, rice, stock, wine and saffron.

3 Cover, bring to a boil, stirring. Simmer, uncovered, for about 35 minutes, stirring occasionally, until almost all the liquid has been absorbed and the rice is tender.

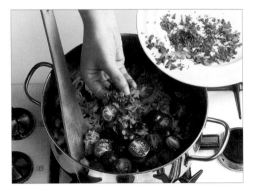

4 Finally, stir in the halved cherry tomatoes. Chop the herbs, and add them to the pan. Season according to taste. Serve the paella immediately, garnished with celery leaves and cherry tomatoes and accompanied by lemon wedges for squeezing.

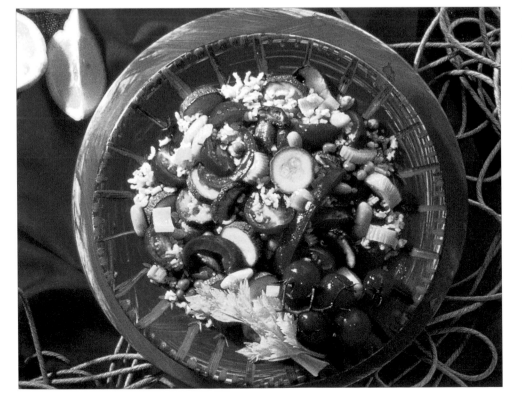

| — NUTRITION NOTES — | |
|---|---|
| Per portion: | |
| Energy | 416kcals |
| Protein | 13.69g |
| Fat | 3.95g |
| Saturated fat | 0.86g |
| Carbohydrate | 84.87g |
| Fiber | 8.85g |
| Added sugar | 0.03g |
| Sodium | 0.54g |

# Vegetable Chili

This vegetarian alternative to traditional chili con carne is particularly good served with brown rice and plain yogurt.

## INGREDIENTS

*Serves 4*

2 onions, chopped
1 garlic clove, crushed
3 celery stalks, chopped
1 green bell pepper, seeded and diced
3 cups mushrooms, sliced
2 zucchini, diced
14-ounce can red kidney beans, rinsed and drained
14-ounce can chopped tomatoes
⅔ cup passata (sieved tomatoes)
2 tablespoons tomato paste
1 tablespoon ketchup
1 teaspoon each hot chili powder, ground cumin and ground coriander
salt and ground black pepper
fresh cilantro sprigs, to garnish
brown rice, plain yogurt and cayenne pepper, to serve

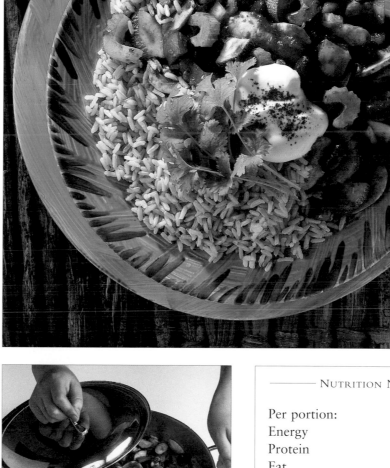

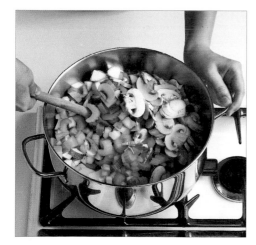

1 Put the onions, garlic, celery, green pepper, mushrooms and zucchini in a large saucepan, and mix together well.

2 Add the kidney beans, tomatoes, passata, tomato paste and ketchup. Stir in the chili powder, cumin, coriander and seasoning, and mix thoroughly.

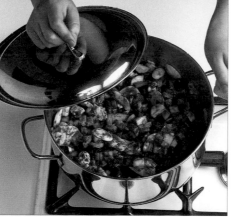

3 Cover, bring to a boil and simmer for 20–30 minutes, stirring occasionally, until the vegetables are tender. Garnish with fresh cilantro sprigs. Serve with brown rice and plain yogurt, sprinkled with cayenne pepper.

| — NUTRITION NOTES — | |
|---|---|
| Per portion: | |
| Energy | 158kcals |
| Protein | 9.96g |
| Fat | 1.59g |
| Saturated fat | 0.27g |
| Carbohydrate | 27.55g |
| Fiber | 8.58g |
| Added sugar | 0.57g |
| Sodium | 0.39g |

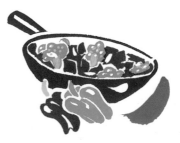

# Cheese, Onion and Mushroom Tart

A flavorful savory tart, this is excellent served with slices of fresh whole-wheat bread and a mixed green salad for extra fiber, vitamins and minerals.

## INGREDIENTS

*Serves 6*

1½ cups whole-wheat flour
a pinch of salt
6 tablespoons polyunsaturated
   margarine
1 onion, sliced
1 leek, sliced
2¼ cups mushrooms, chopped
2 tablespoons vegetable stock
2 eggs
⅔ cup skim milk
4 ounces frozen corn kernels
2 tablespoons snipped fresh chives
1 tablespoon chopped fresh parsley
¾ cup reduced-fat aged
   Cheddar cheese, finely grated
salt and ground black pepper
chives and salad leaves, to garnish

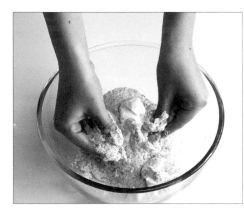

*1* Preheat the oven to 400°F. Sift the flour and salt into a bowl. Rub the fat into the flour, until the mixture resembles bread crumbs.

---COOK'S TIP---

Make this savory tart in advance and freeze for up to three months. Defrost thoroughly, and reheat to serve.

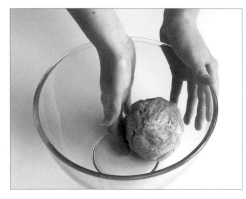

*2* Mix in enough cold water to form a soft, but not sticky, dough. Wrap and chill for 30 minutes.

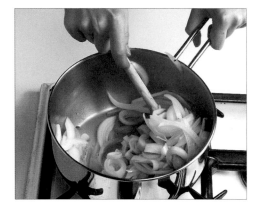

*3* Put the onion and leek into a saucepan. Add the mushrooms and vegetable stock, and bring to a boil. Cover and cook gently for 10 minutes, until the vegetables are tender. Drain.

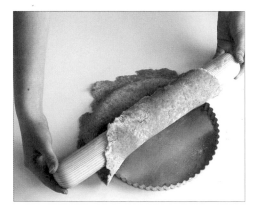

*4* Roll the pastry out on a lightly floured surface and use to line an 8-inch tart pan or dish. Place on a baking sheet.

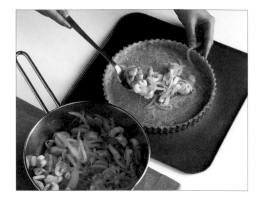

*5* Spoon the vegetables over the pastry. Beat the eggs and milk together, add the corn, herbs, cheese and seasoning, and mix well.

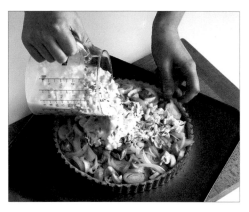

*6* Pour the egg, milk and cheese mixture over the vegetables. Bake for 20 minutes, then reduce the temperature to 350°F, and cook for another 30 minutes, until the tart is set and lightly browned on top. Garnish with chives and salad. Serve either warm or cold, as you prefer.

---NUTRITION NOTES---

Per portion:

| | |
|---|---|
| Energy | 295kcals |
| Protein | 12.75g |
| Fat | 15.52g |
| Saturated fat | 4.10g |
| Carbohydrate | 27.97g |
| Fiber | 4.22g |
| Added sugar | 0.00g |
| Sodium | 0.27g |

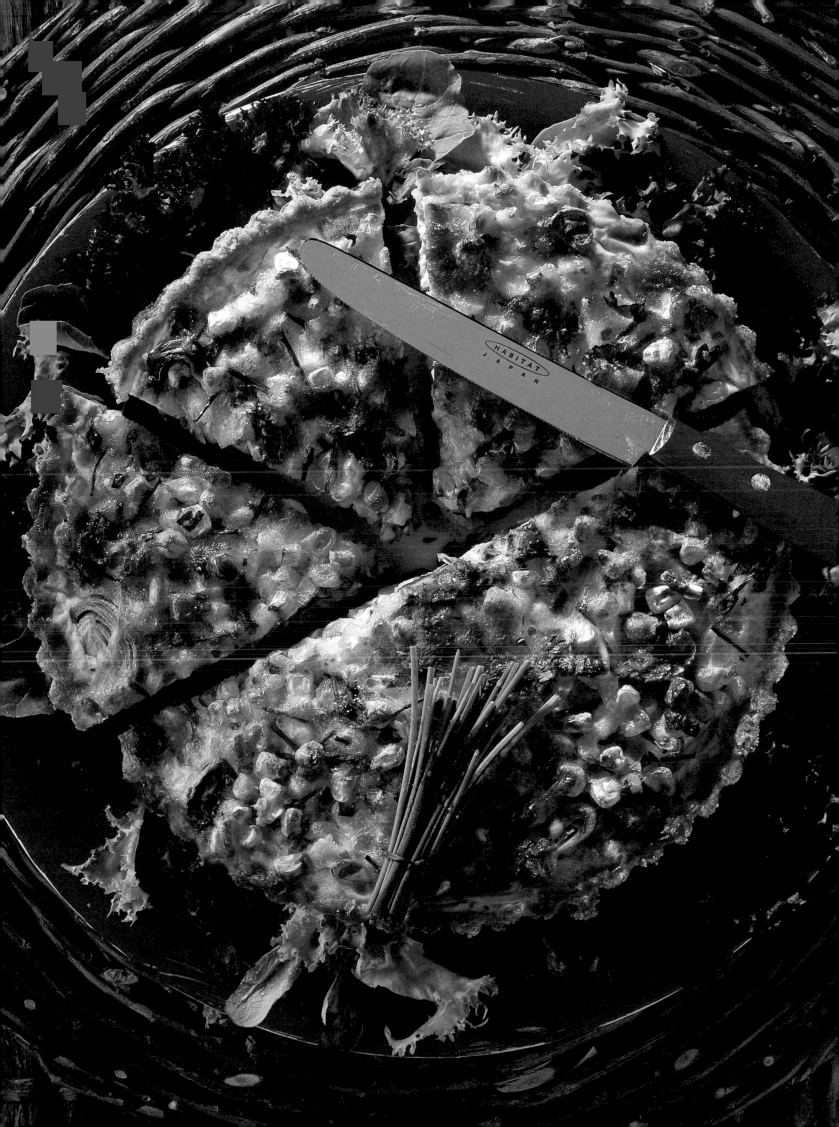

# Sweet-and-Sour Mixed Bean Hot Pot

This appetizing combination of beans and vegetables has a tasty sweet-and-sour sauce, topped with a delicious layer of tender sliced potatoes.

## INGREDIENTS

*Serves 8*

1 pound unpeeled potatoes
1 tablespoon olive oil
3 tablespoons half-fat spread
⅓ cup plain whole-wheat flour
1¼ cups passata (sieved tomatoes)
⅔ cup unsweetened apple juice
4 tablespoons each light brown sugar,
   ketchup, dry sherry, cider vinegar and
   light soy sauce
14-ounce can lima beans
14-ounce can red kidney beans
14-ounce can flageolet beans
14-ounce can chickpeas
6 ounces green beans, chopped
   and blanched
8 ounces shallots, sliced
   and blanched
3 cups mushrooms, sliced
1 tablespoon each chopped fresh thyme
   and marjoram
salt and ground black pepper
fresh herb sprigs, to garnish

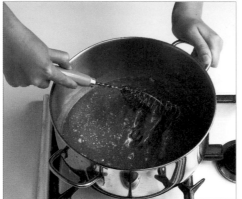

*2* Place the half-fat spread, flour, passata, apple juice, sugar, ketchup, sherry, vinegar and soy sauce in a saucepan. Heat gently, whisking continuously, until the sauce comes to a boil and thickens. Simmer gently for 3 minutes, stirring.

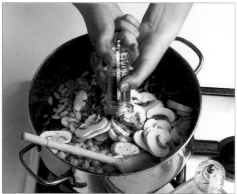

*3* Rinse and drain the canned lima beans, kidney beans, flageolet beans and chickpeas, and add these to the sauce with all the remaining ingredients, except the herb garnish. Mix together well.

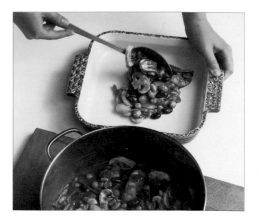

*4* Spoon the bean mixture into a wide casserole.

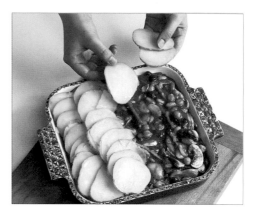

*5* Arrange the potato slices over the top, completely covering the bean mixture.

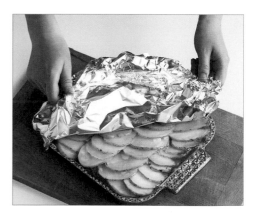

*6* Cover the dish with foil and bake for approximately 1 hour, until the potatoes are cooked and tender. Remove the foil for the last 20 minutes of cooking time to lightly brown the potatoes. Serve immediately, garnished with fresh herb sprigs.

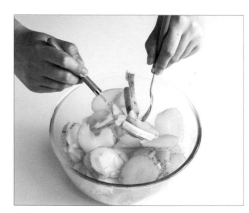

*1* Preheat the oven to 400°F. Thinly slice the potatoes, and parboil them for about 4 minutes. Drain thoroughly, then toss them in the oil so they are lightly coated all over, and set aside.

| NUTRITION NOTES | |
| --- | --- |
| Per portion: | |
| Energy | 410kcals |
| Protein | 17.36g |
| Fat | 7.43g |
| Saturated fat | 1.42g |
| Carbohydrate | 70.40g |
| Fiber | 12.52g |
| Added sugar | 15.86g |
| Sodium | 1.54g |

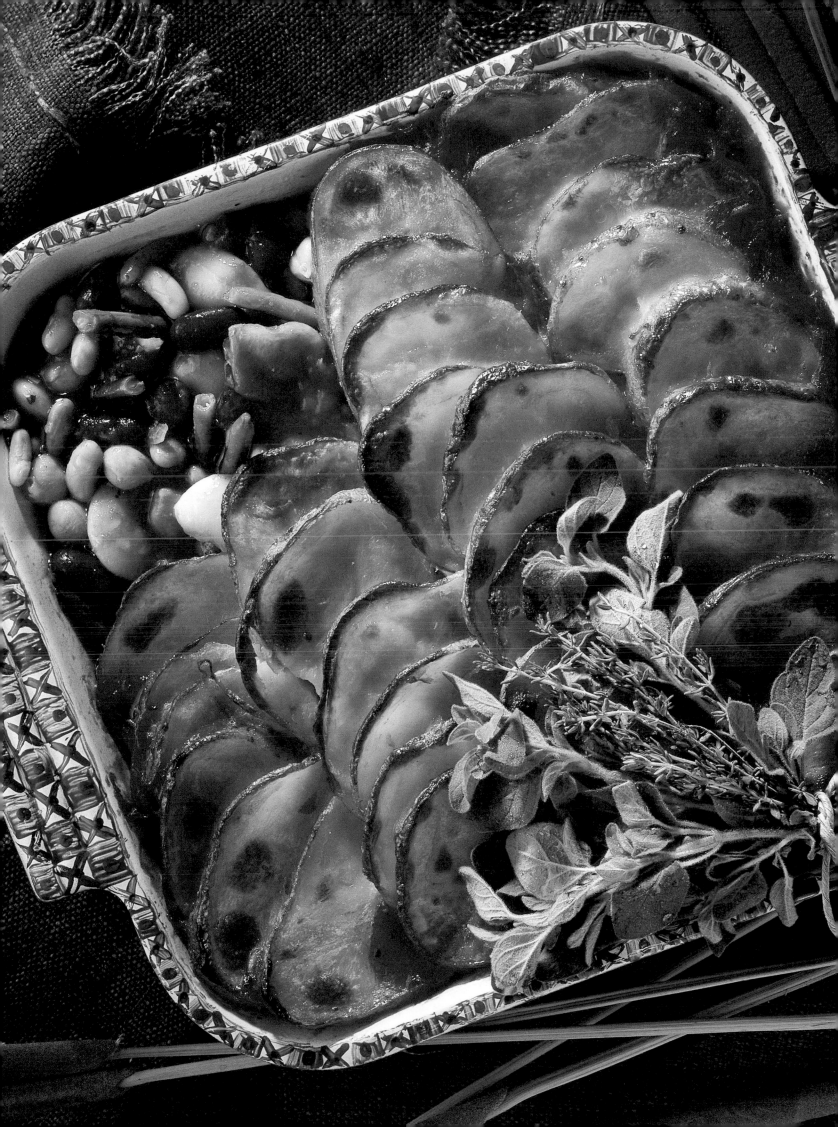

# Zucchini, Corn and Plum Tomato Pizza

This whole-wheat pizza is both healthy and delicious. It can be served hot or cold with a mixed bean salad, and also makes an ideal picnic snack.

## INGREDIENTS

*Serves 6*
2 cups whole-wheat flour
a pinch of salt
2 teaspoons baking powder
4 tablespoons polyunsaturated margarine
⅔ cup skim milk
2 tablespoons tomato paste
2 teaspoons dried herbes de Provence
2 teaspoons olive oil
1 onion, sliced
1 garlic clove, crushed
2 small zucchini, sliced
1½ cups mushrooms, sliced
⅔ cup corn kernels, thawed if frozen
2 plum tomatoes, sliced
½ cup reduced-fat Red Leicester cheese, finely grated
½ cup mozzarella cheese, finely grated
salt and ground black pepper
basil sprigs, to garnish

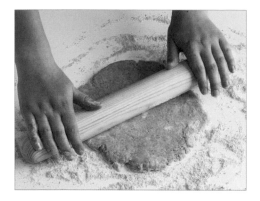

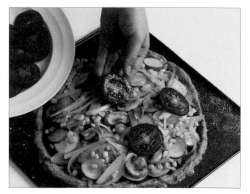

2 Add enough milk to form a soft, but not sticky, dough and knead lightly. Roll the dough out on a lightly floured surface, to a circle about 10 inches in diameter.

5 Spread the prepared vegetable mixture over the pizza crust and sprinkle the corn and seasoning over the top. Then arrange the tomato slices on top.

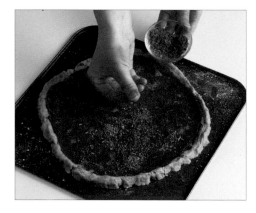

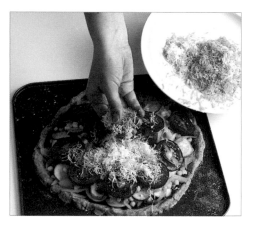

3 Place the dough on the prepared baking sheet, and make the edges slightly thicker than the center. Spread the tomato paste over the crust and sprinkle the herbs on top.

6 Mix together the Red Leicester and mozzarella cheeses and sprinkle them over the pizza. Bake for about 25–30 minutes, until cooked and golden brown on top. Serve the pizza hot or cold in slices, garnished with the basil sprigs.

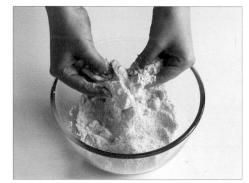

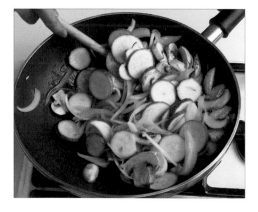

1 Preheat the oven to 425°F. Line a baking sheet with baking parchment. Put the flour, salt and baking powder in a bowl and rub the fat lightly into the flour, until the mixture resembles bread crumbs.

4 Heat the oil in a frying pan, add the onion, garlic, zucchini and mushrooms, and cook gently for 10 minutes, stirring occasionally.

| NUTRITION NOTES | |
| --- | --- |
| Per portion: | |
| Energy | 291kcals |
| Protein | 12.56g |
| Fat | 12.35g |
| Saturated fat | 3.69g |
| Carbohydrate | 34.54g |
| Fiber | 4.93g |
| Added sugar | 0.00g |
| Sodium | 0.25g |

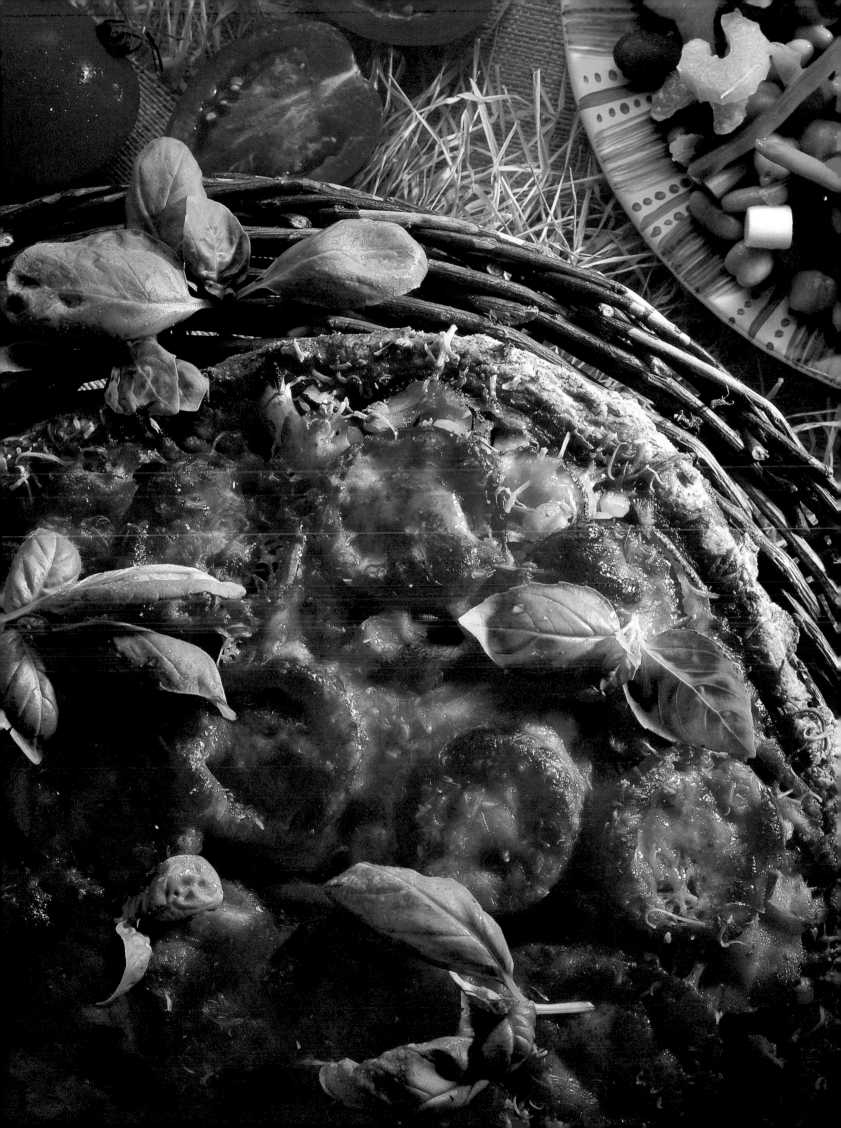

# Vegetable and Macaroni Casserole

A welcome change from macaroni and cheese, this recipe is excellent served with steamed fresh vegetables.

## INGREDIENTS

***Serves 6***

2¼ cups whole-wheat macaroni
2 cups leeks, sliced
3 tablespoons vegetable stock
8 ounces broccoli florets
4 tablespoons half-fat spread
½ cup whole-wheat flour
3⅔ cups skim milk
1¼ cups reduced-fat aged Cheddar
   cheese, grated
1 teaspoon prepared English mustard
12-ounce can corn kernels
½ cup fresh whole-wheat bread crumbs
2 tablespoons chopped fresh parsley
2 tomatoes, cut into eighths
salt and ground black pepper

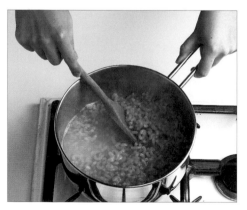

*1* Preheat the oven to 400°F. Cook the macaroni in lightly salted boiling water for about 10 minutes, until just tender, then drain and keep warm.

---

**VARIATION**

Use another reduced-fat hard cheese such as Red Leicester or Double Gloucester in place of the Cheddar cheese.

---

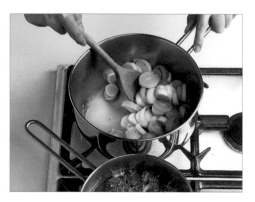

*2* Cook the leeks in the stock for about 10 minutes, until tender, then strain and set aside. Blanch the broccoli in boiling water for 2 minutes, drain and set aside.

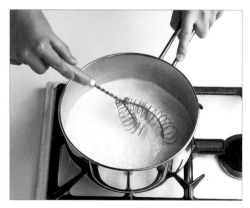

*3* Put the half-fat spread, flour and milk in a saucepan. Heat gently, whisking continuously, until the sauce comes to a boil and thickens. Simmer gently for 3 minutes, stirring.

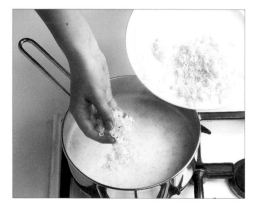

*4* Remove the pan from heat, add 1 cup of the cheese, and stir until it has melted and is well blended with the milk mixture.

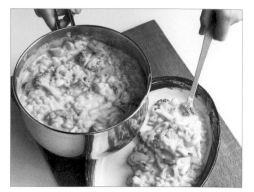

*5* Add the macaroni, leeks, broccoli, mustard, drained corn and seasoning, and mix well. Transfer the mixture to an ovenproof dish.

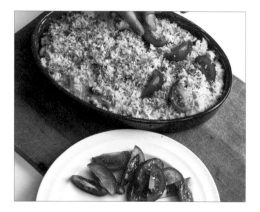

*6* Mix the remaining cheese, bread crumbs and parsley together and sprinkle this mixture over the top. Arrange the tomatoes on top, and then bake for 30–40 minutes, until bubbling and golden brown on top. Serve immediately, while piping hot.

---

**NUTRITION NOTES**

Per portion:
| | |
|---|---|
| Energy | 376kcals |
| Protein | 23.30g |
| Fat | 9.68g |
| Saturated fat | 3.82g |
| Carbohydrate | 52.34g |
| Fiber | 7.12g |
| Added sugar | 0.01g |
| Sodium | 0.53g |

---

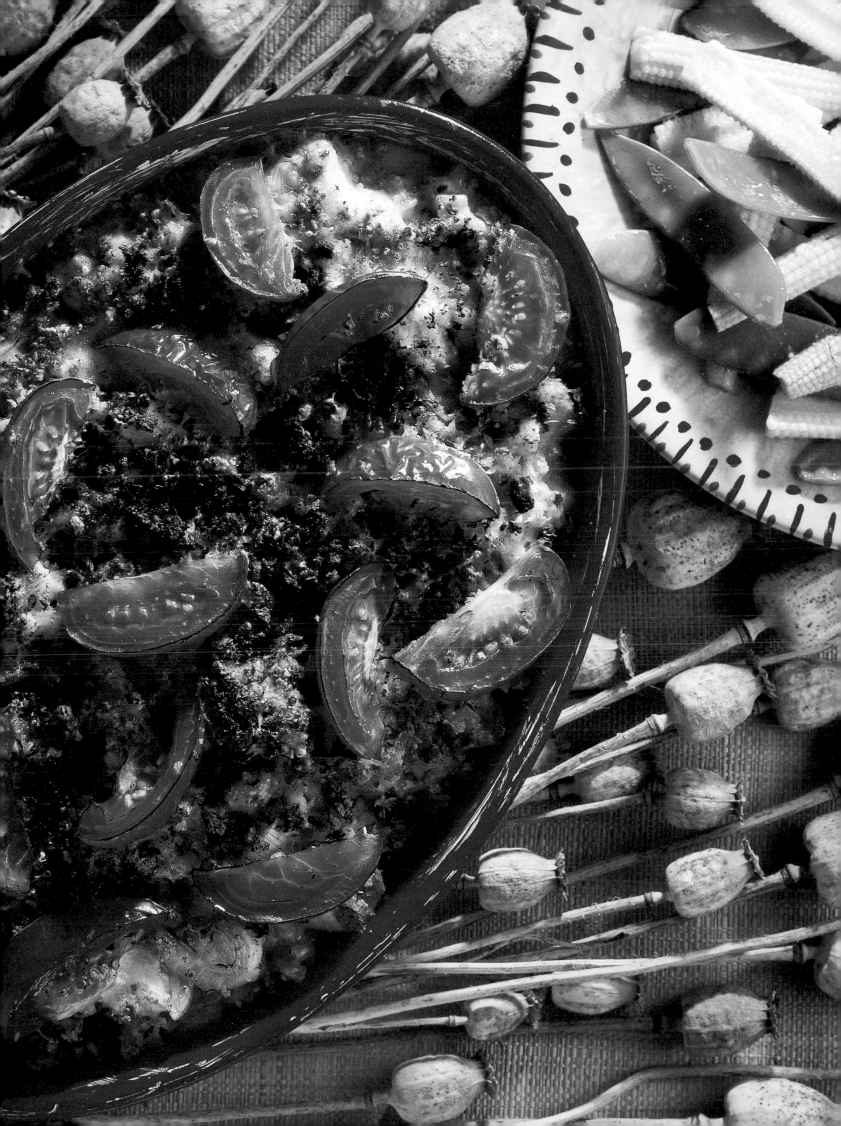

# Curried New Potato and Green Bean Salad

Tender new potatoes and green beans are tossed together in a light, subtly flavored dressing to make this salad. If you want to make a plainer dish, omit the curry paste.

### INGREDIENTS

*Serves 6*

1½ cups green beans, trimmed and
   halved
1½ pounds baby new potatoes, cooked
   in their skins
2 bunches scallions, chopped
¾ cup golden raisins
¾ cup dried pears, finely chopped
6 tablespoons reduced-calorie
   mayonnaise
¼ cup low-fat plain yogurt
2 tablespoons plain yogurt
1 tablespoon tomato paste
1 tablespoon curry paste
2 tablespoons snipped fresh chives
salt and ground black pepper

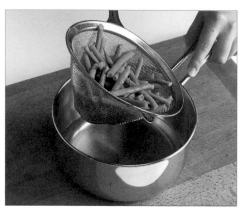

*1* Cook the beans in boiling water for 5 minutes, until tender. Drain, then rinse under cold running water to cool them quickly. Drain again.

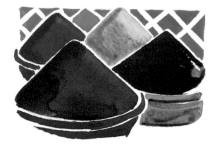

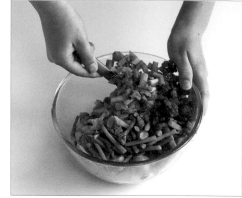

*2* Put the beans, potatoes, scallions, raisins and pears in a bowl, and mix together.

*3* In a small bowl, mix together the mayonnaise, yogurts, tomato paste, curry paste, chives and seasoning.

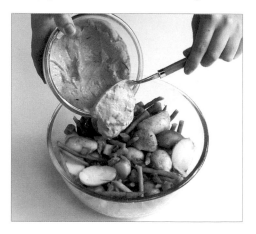

*4* Add the dressing to the vegetables and toss together to mix. Cover and let stand for at least 1 hour before serving, to allow the potatoes to absorb the flavors.

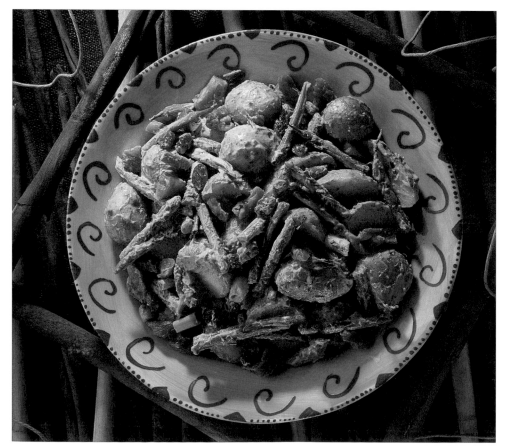

| — NUTRITION NOTES — | |
| --- | --- |
| Per portion: | |
| Energy | 235kcals |
| Protein | 5.17g |
| Fat | 6.10g |
| Saturated fat | 1.06g |
| Carbohydrate | 42.62g |
| Fiber | 3.87g |
| Added sugar | 0.83g |
| Sodium | 0.22g |

# Spicy Bean and Lentil Loaf

This is an unusual meat-free and high-fiber savory loaf, perfect for a picnic.

## INGREDIENTS

*Serves 12*

2 teaspoons olive oil
1 onion, finely chopped
1 garlic clove, crushed
2 celery stalks, finely chopped
14-ounce can red kidney beans
14-ounce can lentils
1 egg
1 carrot, coarsely grated
½ cup hazelnuts, finely chopped
½ cup reduced-fat aged Cheddar
   cheese, finely grated
1 cup fresh whole-wheat bread crumbs
1 tablespoon tomato paste
1 tablespoon ketchup
1 teaspoon each ground cumin, ground
   coriander and hot chili powder
salt and ground black pepper
salad, to serve

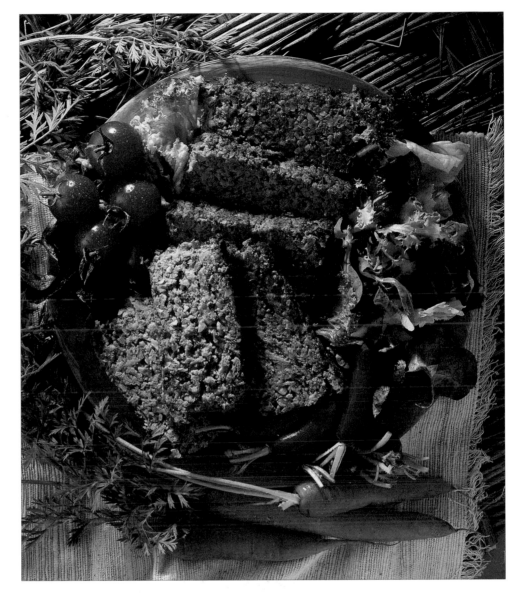

1 Preheat the oven to 350°F. Lightly grease a 9 x 5 x 3-inch loaf pan. Heat the oil in a saucepan, add the onion, garlic and celery and cook for 5 minutes, stirring occasionally. Remove from heat and cool a little.

3 Transfer the bean and lentil mixture to a large bowl, add all the remaining ingredients, and mix well. Season to taste.

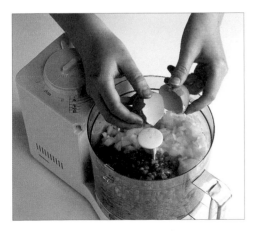

2 Rinse and drain the beans and lentils. Process in a blender or food processor with the onion mixture and egg, until smooth.

| NUTRITION NOTES | |
|---|---|
| Per portion: | |
| Energy | 119kcals |
| Protein | 7.22g |
| Fat | 4.85g |
| Saturated fat | 0.88g |
| Carbohydrate | 12.57g |
| Fiber | 3.31g |
| Added sugar | 0.19g |
| Sodium | 0.17g |

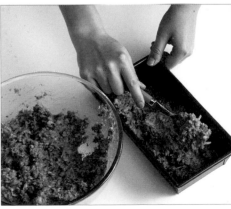

4 Spoon the mixture into the prepared pan and level the surface. Bake for about 1 hour, then remove from the pan and serve hot or cold in slices, accompanied by a salad.

# Fruity Rice Salad

An appetizing and colorful rice salad that combines many different flavors.

## INGREDIENTS

*Serves 4-6*

1 cup mixed brown and wild rice
1 yellow bell pepper, seeded and diced
1 bunch scallions, chopped
3 celery stalks, chopped
1 large beefsteak tomato, chopped
2 Granny Smith apples, chopped
¾ cup dried apricots, chopped
¾ cup raisins
2 tablespoons unsweetened
    apple juice
2 tablespoons dry sherry
2 tablespoons light soy sauce
dash of Tabasco sauce
2 tablespoons chopped fresh parsley
1 tablespoon chopped fresh rosemary
salt and ground black pepper

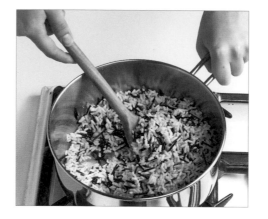

*1* Cook the rice in a large saucepan of lightly salted boiling water for about 30 minutes (or according to the instructions on the package), until tender. Rinse the rice under cold running water to cool quickly, and then drain thoroughly.

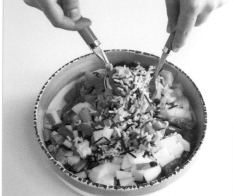

*2* Place the yellow pepper, scallions, celery, tomato, apples, apricots, raisins and the cooked rice in a serving bowl, and mix well.

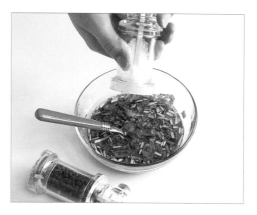

*3* In a small bowl, mix together the apple juice, sherry, soy sauce, Tabasco sauce, herbs and seasoning.

*4* Pour the dressing over the rice mixture and toss the ingredients together to mix. Serve immediately, or cover and chill in the refrigerator before serving.

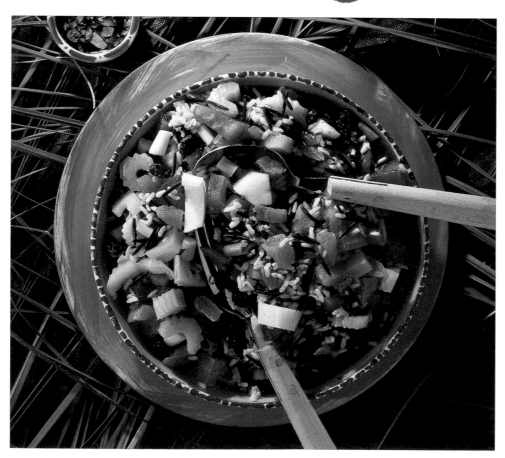

| NUTRITION NOTES | |
| --- | --- |
| Per portion: | |
| Energy | 428kcals |
| Protein | 8.15g |
| Fat | 2.50g |
| Saturated fat | 0.52g |
| Carbohydrate | 97.15g |
| Fiber | 7.17g |
| Added sugar | 0.31g |
| Sodium | 0.58g |

# Bulgur and Fava Bean Salad

This summery salad is perfect served with fresh, crusty whole-wheat bread and homemade chutney or relish. For non-vegetarians, it can be served as an accompaniment to broiled lean meat or fish.

## INGREDIENTS

*Serves 6*

2 cups bulgur
8 ounces frozen fava or lima beans
1 cup frozen tiny peas
8 ounces cherry tomatoes, halved
1 sweet onion, chopped
1 red bell pepper, seeded and diced
2 ounces snow peas, chopped
2 ounces watercress
1 tablespoon chopped fresh parsley
1 tablespoon chopped fresh basil
1 tablespoon chopped fresh thyme
fat-free French dressing
salt and ground black pepper

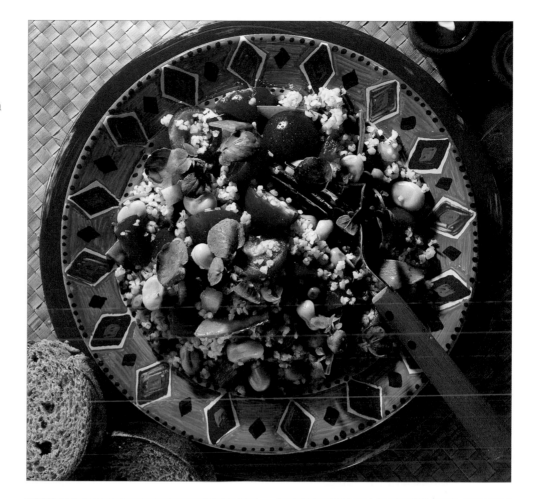

*1* Soak and cook the bulgur according to the package instructions. Drain thoroughly, and put into a serving bowl.

*2* Meanwhile, cook the frozen beans and peas in lightly salted, boiling water for approximately 3 minutes, until tender. Drain them thoroughly, and add to the prepared bulgur.

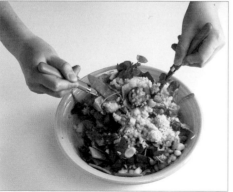

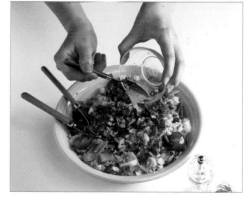

*3* Add the cherry tomatoes, onion, pepper, snow peas and watercress to the bulgur mixture and mix.

*4* Add the herbs, seasoning and French dressing to taste, tossing the ingredients together. Serve immediately, or cover and chill before serving.

| NUTRITION NOTES | |
| --- | --- |
| Per portion: | |
| Energy | 277kcals |
| Protein | 11.13g |
| Fat | 1.81g |
| Saturated fat | 0.17g |
| Carbohydrate | 55.34g |
| Fiber | 4.88g |
| Added sugar | 0.00g |
| Sodium | 0.02g |

### VARIATION

Use cooked couscous, boiled brown rice or whole-wheat pasta in place of the bulgur, if you prefer.

# Roasted Bell Pepper and Wild Mushroom Pasta Salad

This pasta salad is colorful as well as highly nutritious.

## INGREDIENTS

*Serves 6*
1 red bell pepper, halved
1 yellow bell pepper, halved
1 green bell pepper, halved
3 cups whole-wheat pasta
  shells or twists
2 tablespoons olive oil
3 tablespoons balsamic vinegar
5 tablespoons tomato juice
2 tablespoons chopped fresh basil
1 tablespoon chopped fresh thyme
2⅓ cups shiitake mushrooms, sliced
2⅓ cups oyster mushrooms, sliced
14-ounce can black-eyed beans, rinsed
  and drained
¾ cup golden raisins
2 bunches scallions,
  finely chopped
salt and ground black pepper

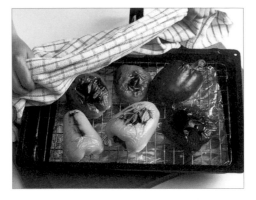

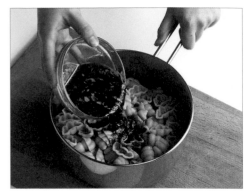

1 Preheat the broiler. Put the halved red and yellow bell peppers cut side down on a broiler pan rack, and place under a hot broiler for 10–15 minutes, until the skins are charred. Cover the peppers with a clean, damp dish towel, and set aside to cool.

2 Meanwhile, cook the whole-wheat pasta shells or twists in lightly salted boiling water for 10–12 minutes (or according to the instructions on the package), until al dente, then drain thoroughly.

3 Mix together the oil, vinegar, tomato juice, basil and thyme, add to the warm pasta, and toss together.

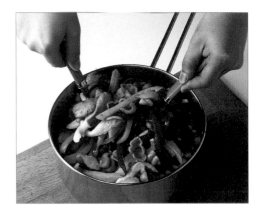

4 Remove and discard the skins from the bell peppers; they should come away easily. Seed and slice the peppers, and add to the pasta along with the mushrooms, beans, raisins, scallions and seasoning. Toss all the ingredients together in the bowl to mix well, and serve immediately. Alternatively, cover the salad bowl, and chill in the refrigerator for several hours before serving.

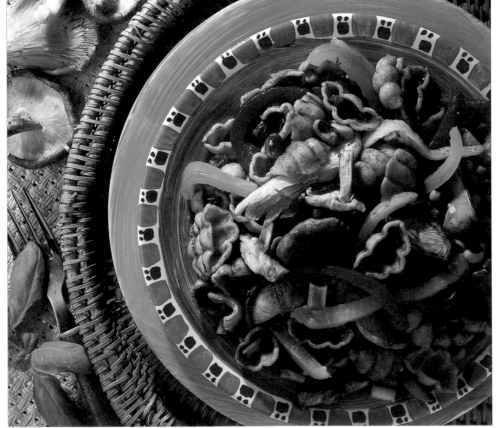

| NUTRITION NOTES | |
| --- | --- |
| Per portion: | |
| Energy | 334kcals |
| Protein | 13.58g |
| Fat | 6.02g |
| Saturated fat | 0.89g |
| Carbohydrate | 60.74g |
| Fiber | 9.37g |
| Added sugar | 0.00g |
| Sodium | 0.11g |

# Carrot, Raisin and Apricot Coleslaw

This is a high-fiber coleslaw, combining cabbage, carrots and dried fruit in a nutritious light yogurt dressing.

## INGREDIENTS

*Serves 6*

3 cups white cabbage, finely shredded
1½ cups carrots, coarsely grated
1 red onion, sliced
3 celery stalks, sliced
1 cup raisins
⅓ cup dried apricots, chopped
½ cup reduced-calorie mayonnaise
6 tablespoons low-fat plain yogurt
2 tablespoons chopped fresh
  mixed herbs
salt and ground black pepper

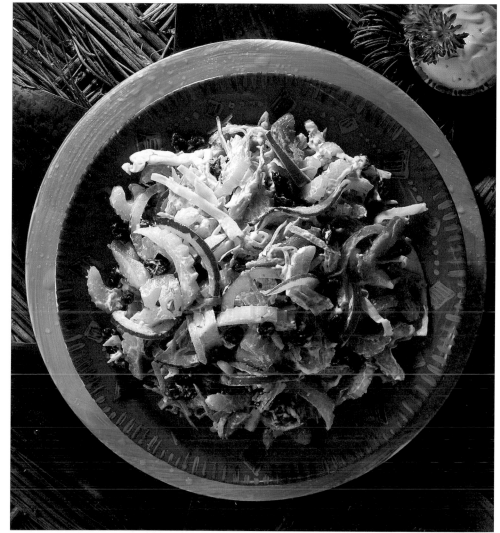

*1* Put the cabbage and carrots in a large bowl.

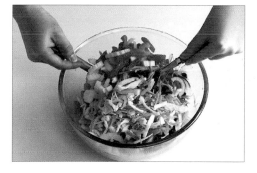

*2* Add the onion, celery, raisins and apricots, and mix well.

### NUTRITION NOTES

Per portion:

| | |
|---|---|
| Energy | 204kcals |
| Protein | 3.71g |
| Fat | 6.37g |
| Saturated fat | 0.93g |
| Carbohydrate | 35.04g |
| Fiber | 4.25g |
| Added sugar | 0.50g |
| Sodium | 0.24g |

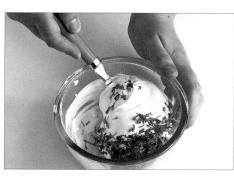

*3* In a small bowl, mix together the mayonnaise, yogurt, fresh herbs and seasoning.

### VARIATION

Use other dried fruit such as golden raisins and dried pears or peaches instead of the raisins and apricots.

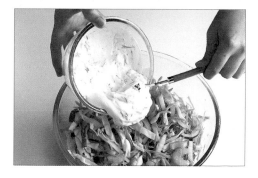

*4* Add the mayonnaise dressing to the bowl, and toss the ingredients together to mix. Cover and chill for several hours before serving.

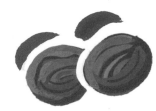

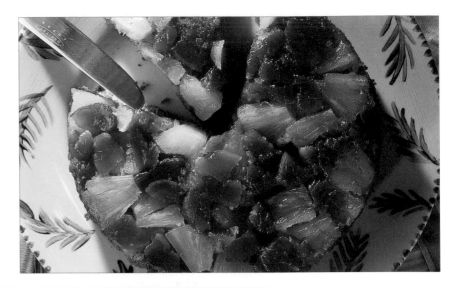

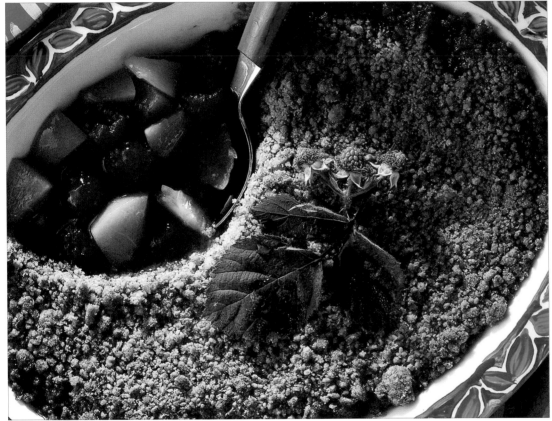

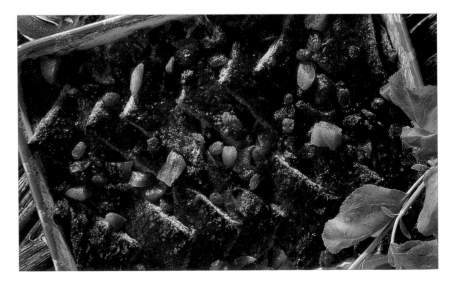

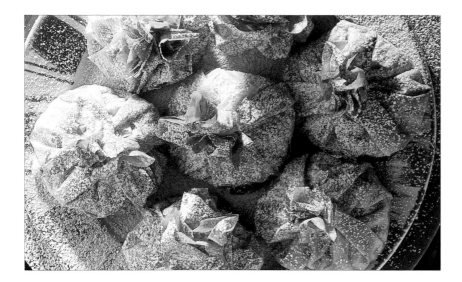

# HOT AND COLD DESSERTS

*Delectable desserts are always tempting, but this does not mean that they need to be too unhealthy. There are plenty of ways to increase the fiber content of puddings and desserts. Fruit, whether fresh, dried or cooked, combines deliciously with whole-wheat flours and whole-wheat breads to make sweet treats such as Pineapple and Peach Upside-down Pudding or Peach and Raspberry Crumble. Such winter warmers are satisfying but may be somewhat substantial for sizzling summer days. If you prefer something light and luscious, try Tropical Fruit Phyllo Clusters or a scoop of Whole-wheat Bread and Banana Yogurt Ice, which is a lot lighter than its name suggests. A mixture of dried and fresh fruit makes a superb sweet salad, as demonstrated by Apricot and Banana Compote, which is equally suitable for breakfast or after dinner.*

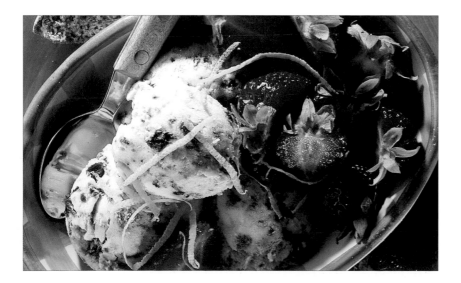

# Pineapple and Peach Upside-down Pudding

An inspired combination of pineapple and peaches, this old favorite goes well with ice cream or even low-fat custard, for a healthier alternative. It is also a lot of fun to make.

### INGREDIENTS

*Serves 6*

5 tablespoons golden or light
  corn syrup
8-ounce can pineapple chunks in
  fruit juice
¾ cup dried peaches, chopped
⅔ cup sugar
½ cup half-fat spread
1½ cups whole-wheat flour
1½ teaspoons baking powder
½ teaspoon salt
2 eggs

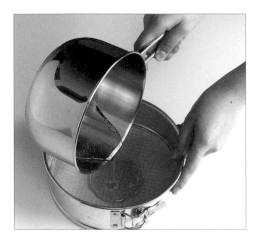

*2* Heat the syrup gently in a saucepan, and pour over the bottom of the pan.

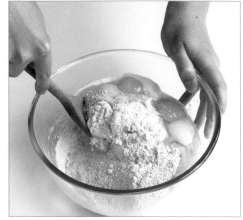

*5* Put the sugar, half-fat spread, flour, baking powder, eggs and reserved pineapple juice in a bowl and beat together until smooth.

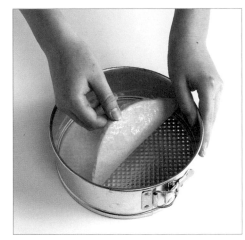

*1* Preheat the oven to 350°F. Lightly grease a loose-bottomed 7-inch round cake pan and line the bottom with baking parchment.

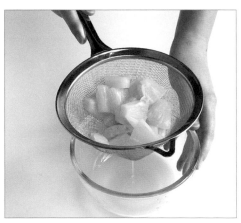

*3* Strain the pineapple, reserving 3 tablespoons of the juice.

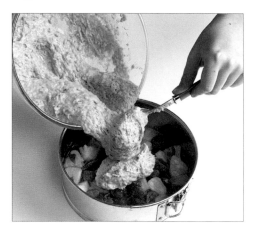

*6* Spread the pudding mixture evenly over the fruit and level the surface. Bake for about 45 minutes, until risen and golden brown. Turn out carefully onto a serving plate and serve hot or cold in slices.

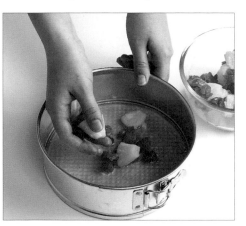

*4* Mix together the pineapple and peaches, and scatter them over the syrup layer in the pan.

--- NUTRITION NOTES ---

| Per portion: | |
| --- | --- |
| Energy | 410kcals |
| Protein | 8.36g |
| Fat | 10.69g |
| Saturated fat | 2.82g |
| Carbohydrate | 74.73g |
| Fiber | 4.94g |
| Added sugar | 37.51g |
| Sodium | 0.21g |

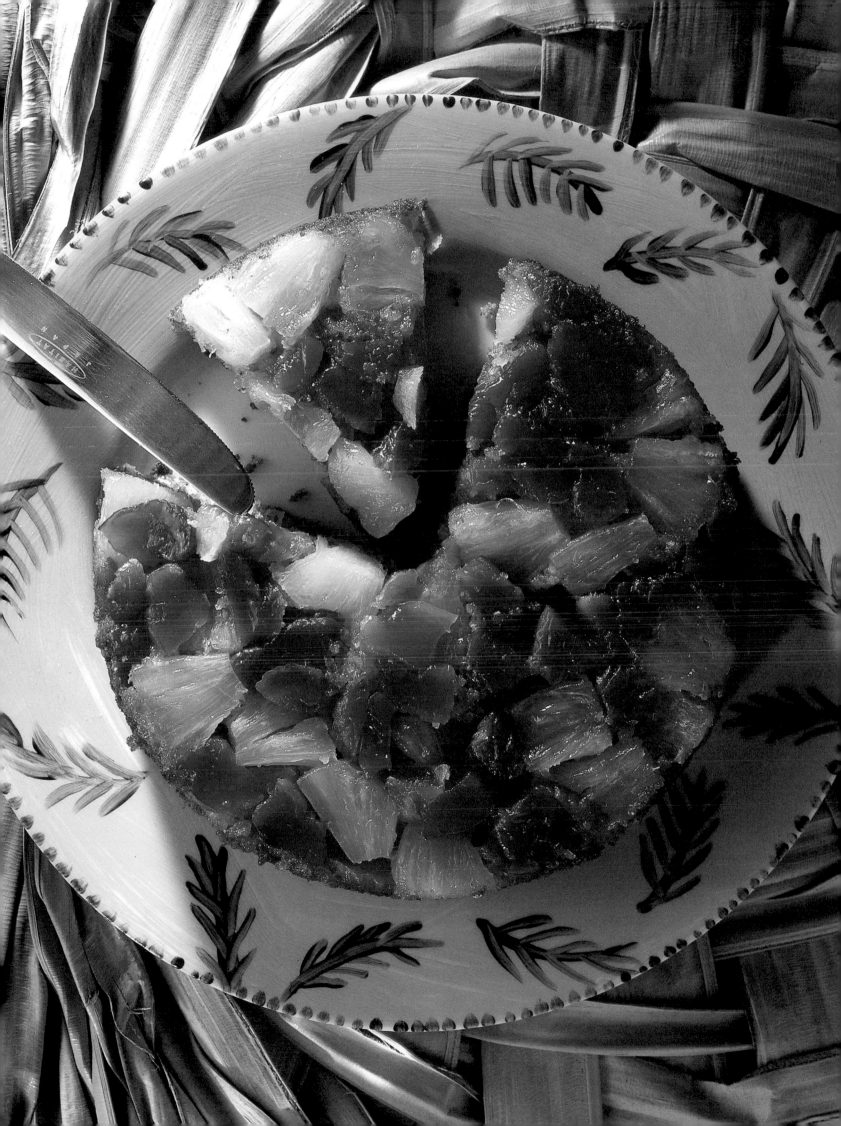

# Peach and Raspberry Crumble

A scrumptious, quick and easy dessert, this crumble is good served hot or cold, on its own or with cream or yogurt.

### INGREDIENTS

*Serves 4*
⅔ cup whole-wheat flour
¾ cup medium oatmeal
6 tablespoons half-fat spread
¼ cup light brown sugar
½ teaspoon ground cinnamon
14-ounce can peach slices in
  fruit juice
1⅓ cups raspberries
2 tablespoons honey
raspberry leaves, to decorate

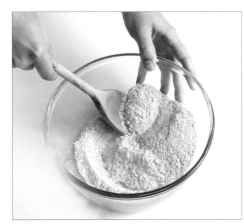

*1* Preheat the oven to 350°F. Put the flour and oatmeal in a bowl, and mix together.

---
VARIATION
---
Use other combinations of fruits, depending on what is available.

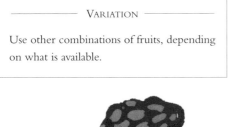
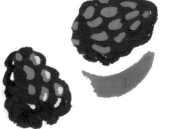

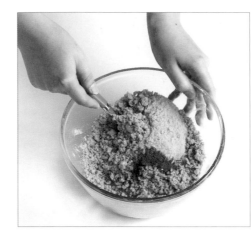

*2* Rub in the half-fat spread until the mixture resembles bread crumbs, then stir in the sugar and cinnamon.

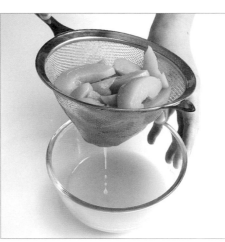

*3* Drain the peach slices and reserve the juice.

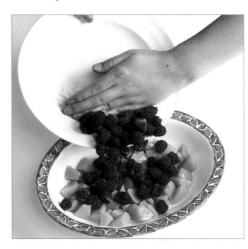

*4* Roughly chop the peaches and put them in an ovenproof dish, then scatter the raspberries over them.

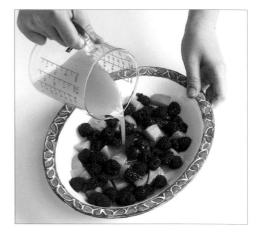

*5* Mix together the reserved peach juice and honey, pour over the fruit and stir.

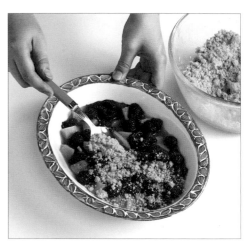

*6* Spoon the crumble mixture over the fruit, pressing it down lightly. Bake for about 45 minutes, until golden brown on top. Serve hot or cold, as you prefer, decorated with raspberry leaves.

---
NUTRITION NOTES
---
Per portion:
| | |
|---|---|
| Energy | 334kcals |
| Protein | 7.02g |
| Fat | 9.9g |
| Saturated fat | 2.51g |
| Carbohydrate | 58.57g |
| Fiber | 5.22g |
| Added sugar | 12.66g |
| Sodium | 0.14g |

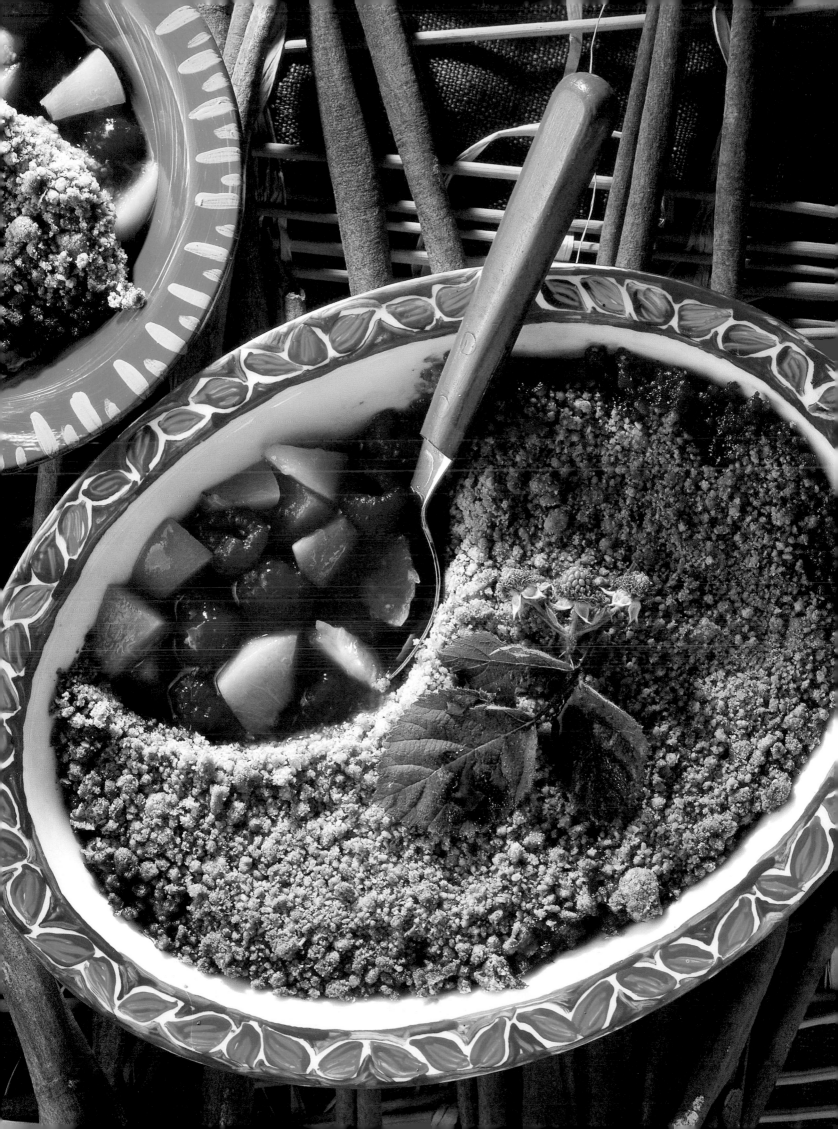

# Fruit and Spice Bread Pudding

An easy-to-make fruity dessert with a hint of spice, this is a healthier, more fiber-rich version of the traditional pudding.

### INGREDIENTS

*Serves 4*
6 medium slices whole-wheat bread
2 ounces reduced-sugar jam
⅓ cup golden raisins
¼ cup dried apricots, chopped
¼ cup light brown sugar
1 teaspoon pumpkin pie spice
2 eggs
2½ cups skim milk
finely grated zest of 1 lemon

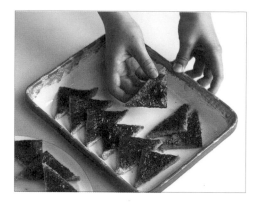

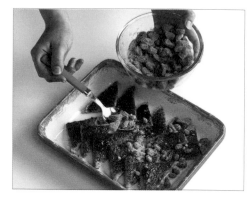

*1* Preheat the oven to 325°F. Remove and discard the crusts from the slices of whole-wheat bread. Spread the bread slices with a jam of your choice, and cut them into small triangles. Place half the bread triangles in two long columns in a lightly greased ovenproof dish.

*2* Mix together the raisins, apricots, sugar and spice, and sprinkle half the fruit mixture evenly over the bread in the dish.

*3* Top with the remaining bread triangles, and then sprinkle the remaining fruit mixture over.

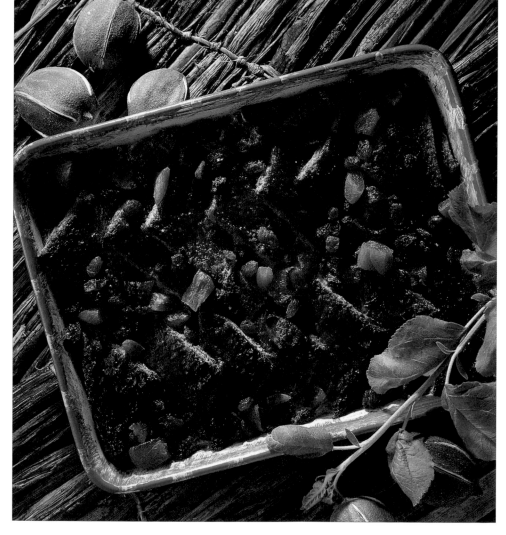

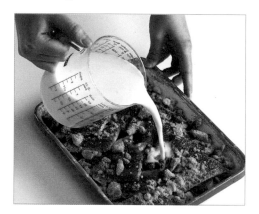

*4* Beat the eggs, milk and lemon zest together in a bowl, and pour over the bread. Set aside for 30 minutes to allow the bread to absorb some of the liquid. Bake for 45–60 minutes, until set and golden brown. Serve hot or cold.

| NUTRITION NOTES | |
| --- | --- |
| Per portion: | |
| Energy | 305kcals |
| Protein | 13.77g |
| Fat | 4.51g |
| Saturated fat | 1.27g |
| Carbohydrate | 56.38g |
| Fiber | 3.75g |
| Added sugar | 13.47g |
| Sodium | 0.38g |

# Apricot and Banana Compote

This compote is delicious served on its own or with custard or ice cream. Served for breakfast with yogurt, it makes a tasty and nutritious start to the day.

### INGREDIENTS

*Serves 4*

1 cup dried apricots
1¼ cups unsweetened orange juice
⅔ cup unsweetened apple juice
1 teaspoon ground ginger
3 medium bananas
¼ cup toasted sliced almonds

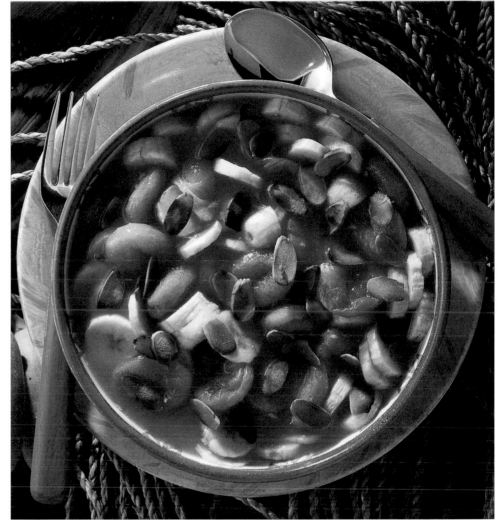

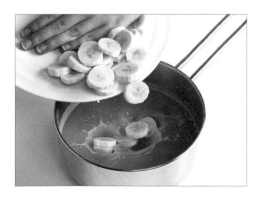

*1* Put the apricots in a saucepan with the fruit juices and ginger and stir. Cover, bring to a boil and simmer gently for 10 minutes, stirring from time to time.

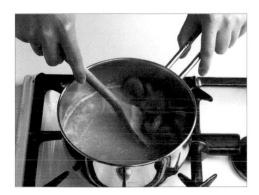

*2* Set aside to cool, leaving the lid on. Slice the bananas into thick slices, and stir them into the cooled cooked apricot mixture.

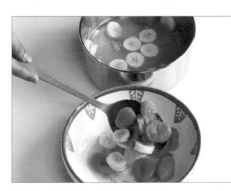

*3* Spoon the fruit and juices into a serving dish.

---
### VARIATION

Use other combinations of dried and fresh fruit such as prunes, figs, apples or peaches.

---

*4* Serve this compote immediately, or cover and chill for several hours in the refrigerator before serving. Sprinkle with toasted sliced almonds, to serve.

---
### NUTRITION NOTES

Per portion:

| | |
|---|---|
| Energy | 241kcals |
| Protein | 4.92g |
| Fat | 4.18g |
| Saturated fat | 0.37g |
| Carbohydrate | 48.98g |
| Fiber | 4.91g |
| Added sugar | 0.00g |
| Sodium | 0.02g |

# Tropical Fruit Phyllo Clusters

These fruity phyllo clusters make a great family treat or dinner-party dessert. They are delicious served hot or cold, either on their own or with cream.

## INGREDIENTS

*Makes 8*

1 banana, peeled and sliced
1 small mango, peeled, pitted and diced
lemon juice, to sprinkle
1 small cooking apple, coarsely grated
6 fresh or dried dates, pitted and chopped
2 ounces dried pineapple, chopped
⅓ cup golden raisins
¼ cup light brown sugar
1 teaspoon pumpkin pie spice
8 sheets phyllo pastry
2 tablespoons sunflower oil
confectioners' sugar, to serve

---

## NUTRITION NOTES

Per portion:

| | |
|---|---|
| Energy | 197kcals |
| Protein | 3.09g |
| Fat | 3.58g |
| Saturated fat | 0.44g |
| Carbohydrate | 40.21g |
| Fiber | 2.31g |
| Added sugar | 9.96g |
| Sodium | 0.16g |

---

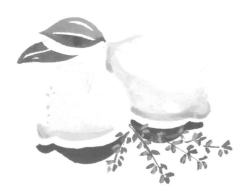

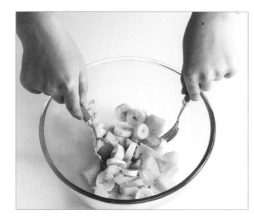

*1* Preheat the oven to 400°F. Line a baking sheet with baking parchment. Toss the banana and mango in lemon juice to prevent discoloration.

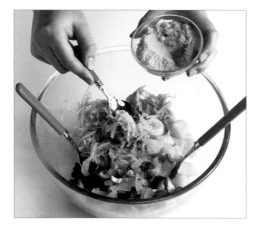

*2* Add the apple, dates, pineapple, raisins, sugar and spice, and mix.

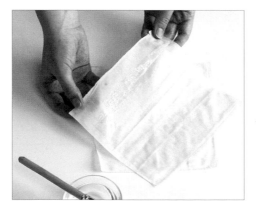

*3* For the clusters, cut each sheet of phyllo pastry in half. Cover when not in use to keep moist. Lightly brush the two squares of pastry with oil, and place one on top of the other at a 90° angle.

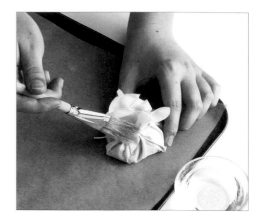

*4* Spoon some fruit filling into the center, gather the pastry up over the filling, and secure with string. Place the cluster on the prepared baking sheet, and lightly brush all over with oil.

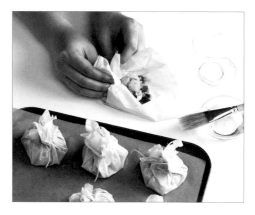

*5* Repeat with the remaining ingredients to make a total of eight fruit clusters. Bake for 25–30 minutes, until golden brown and crisp.

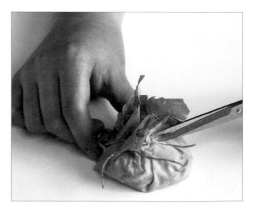

*6* Carefully snip and discard the string from each cluster. Serve the clusters hot or cold, dusted with sifted confectioners' sugar.

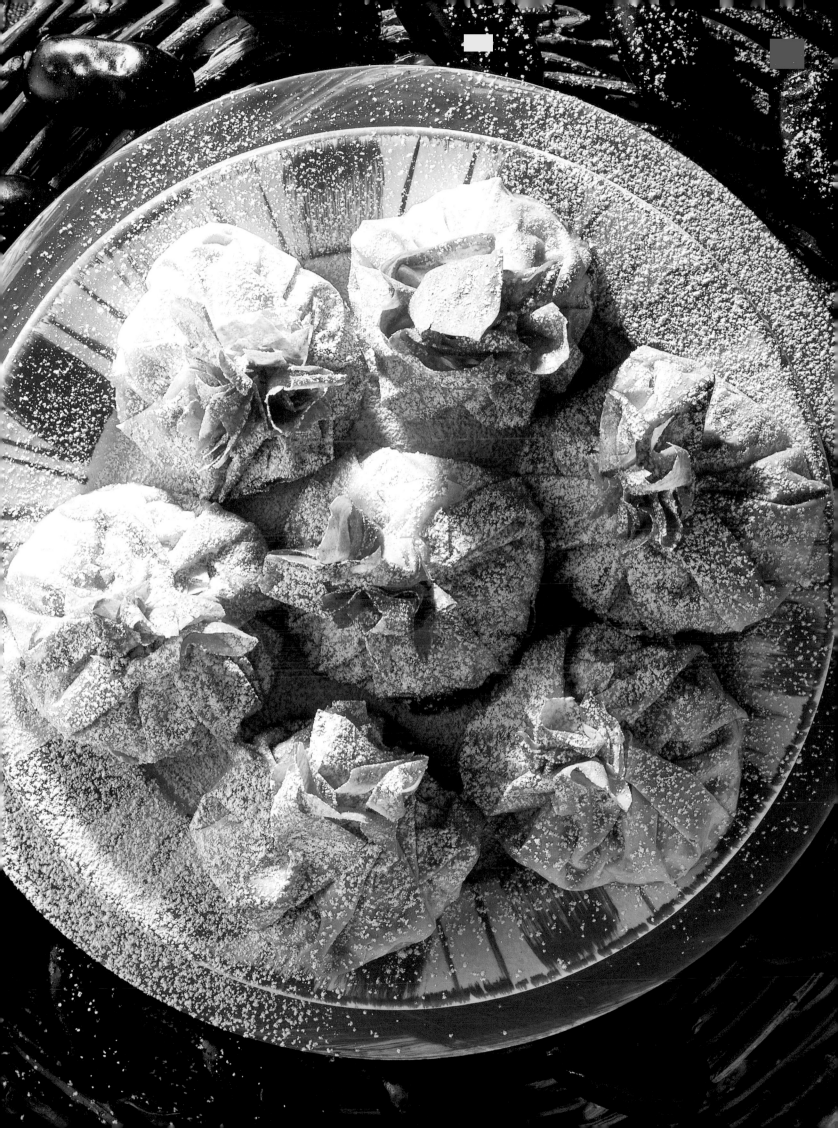

# Winter Fruit Salad

A colorful, refreshing and nutritious fruit salad, which is wonderful served with plain yogurt or cream.

## INGREDIENTS

### Serves 6

8-ounce can pineapple chunks in
   fruit juice
scant 1 cup freshly squeezed
   orange juice
scant 1 cup unsweetened apple juice
2 tablespoons orange or apple liqueur
2 tablespoons honey (optional)
2 oranges, peeled
2 green apples, peeled and sliced
2 pears, peeled and sliced
4 plums, pitted and sliced
12 fresh dates, pitted and chopped
½ cup dried apricots, sliced
1 fresh mint sprig, to decorate

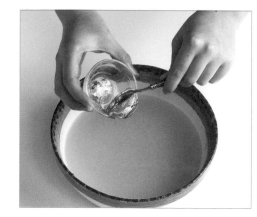

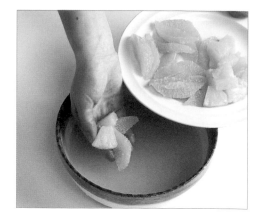

*1* Drain the pineapple, reserving the juice. Put the juice from the pineapple, the orange juice, apple juice, liqueur and honey, if using, in a large serving bowl, and stir to mix.

---

#### VARIATION

Use other unsweetened fruit juices such as pink grapefruit and pineapple juice in place of the orange and apple juice.

---

*2* Segment the oranges, catching any juice in the bowl, and put the orange segments and pineapple into the fruit juice mixture.

*3* Add the apples and pears to the bowl, and mix well.

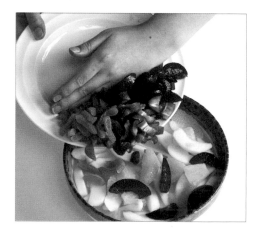

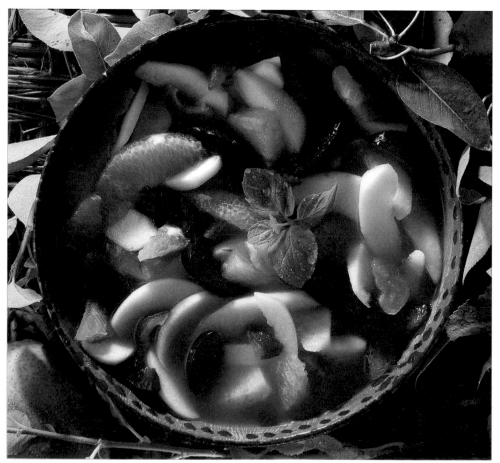

*4* Stir in the plums, dates and apricots, cover and chill for several hours. Decorate with a fresh mint sprig before serving.

---

#### NUTRITION NOTES

Per portion:

| | |
|---|---|
| Energy | 227kcals |
| Protein | 2.85g |
| Fat | 0.37g |
| Saturated fat | 0.00g |
| Carbohydrate | 53.68g |
| Fiber | 5.34g |
| Added sugar | 1.33g |
| Sodium | 0.01g |

# Whole-wheat Bread and Banana Yogurt Ice

Serve this tempting yogurt ice with seasonal fresh fruit and some wafer cookies for a tasty, light dessert.

## INGREDIENTS

*Serves 6*

2 cups fresh whole-wheat bread crumbs
¼ cup light brown sugar
1¼ cups cold low-fat custard
generous 1 cup low-fat fromage frais
generous 1 cup plain yogurt
4 bananas
juice of 1 lemon
¼ cup confectioners' sugar, sifted
⅓ cup raisins, chopped
pared lemon zest, to decorate
strawberries and cookies, to serve

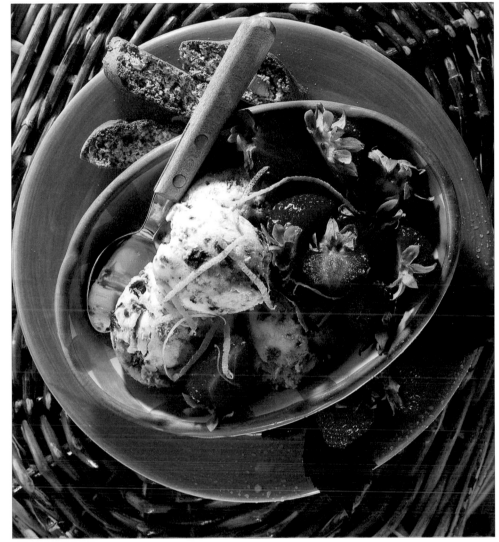

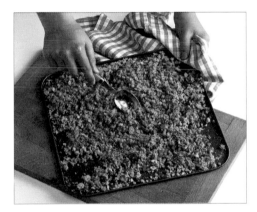

1 Preheat the oven to 400°F. Mix together the bread crumbs and brown sugar, and spread the mixture out on a nonstick baking sheet. Bake for about 10 minutes, until crisp, stirring occasionally. Set aside to cool, then break the mixture up into crumbs.

2 Meanwhile, put the custard, fromage frais and yogurt in a bowl, and mix thoroughly. Mash the bananas with the lemon juice, and add to the custard mixture, stirring well. Fold in the confectioners' sugar.

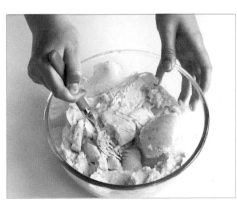

3 Pour the mixture into a shallow, freezerproof container and let freeze for about 3 hours, or until the mixture has become mushy in consistency. Spoon into a chilled bowl and quickly mash the chunks up with a fork, in order to break down the ice crystals.

4 Add the bread crumbs and raisins, and mix well. Return the mixture to the container, cover and freeze until firm. Transfer to the refrigerator 30 minutes before serving, to soften a little. Decorate with lemon zest and serve with strawberries and cookies.

| NUTRITION NOTES | |
| --- | --- |
| Per portion: | |
| Energy | 277kcals |
| Protein | 7.55g |
| Fat | 5.51g |
| Saturated fat | 2.99g |
| Carbohydrate | 52.27g |
| Fiber | 2.01g |
| Added sugar | 12.77g |
| Sodium | 0.17g |

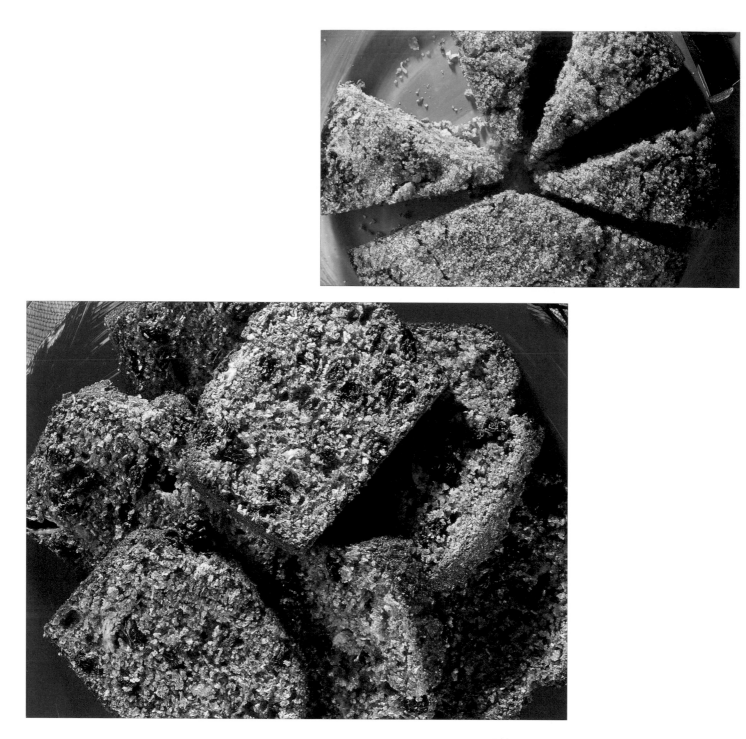
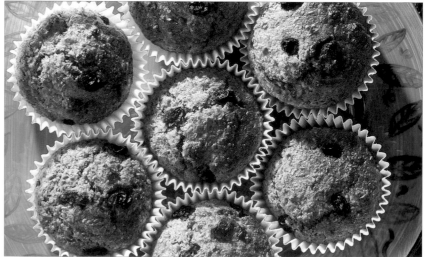

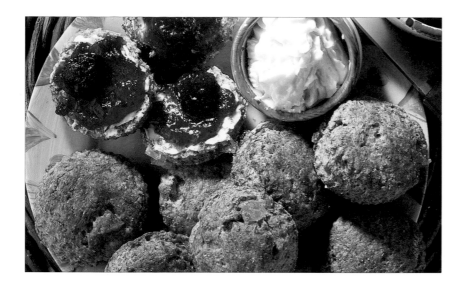

# BAKED GOODS

*Bran is the obvious ingredient for boosting the fiber content of cakes and other baked goods, but it is by no means the only candidate. Although Pear and Golden Raisin Bran Muffins and Banana Bran Loaf are both temptingly tasty, Carrot and Coconut Cake has more fiber per portion than either and is beautifully moist and flavorful. Another moist and fruity choice is Farmhouse Apple and Golden Raisin Cake, while Date and Orange Slices are gloriously chewy and popular with children. On the savory front, try Cheese and Herb Whole-wheat Soda Bread or, for an afternoon snack, enjoy Cheese and Pineapple Whole-wheat Scones. Both are delicious toasted and served with low-fat spread.*

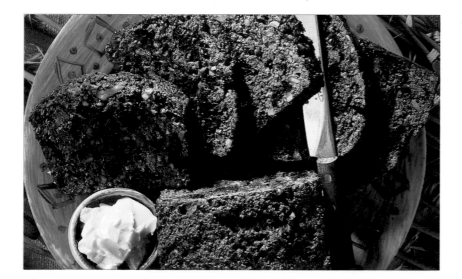

# Pear and Golden Raisin Bran Muffins

These mouthwatering muffins are a real delight. They are best eaten freshly baked and perhaps spread with a little butter or low-fat spread and honey.

## INGREDIENTS

*Makes 12*

⅔ cup whole-wheat
  flour, sifted
½ cup all-purpose
  flour, sifted
2½ cups bran
1 tablespoon baking
  powder, sifted
pinch of salt
4 tablespoons half-fat spread
¼ cup light brown sugar
1 egg
scant 1 cup skim milk
½ cup dried pears, chopped
⅓ cup golden raisins

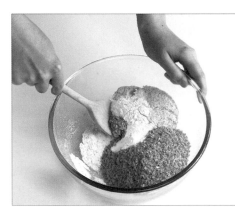

*1* Preheat the oven to 400°F. Lightly grease 12 muffin or deep-cup bun pans or line them with paper muffin cases. Mix together the whole-wheat and all-purpose flours, bran, baking powder and salt in a bowl.

---

COOK'S TIP

For a quick and easy way to chop dried fruit, snip with kitchen scissors.

---

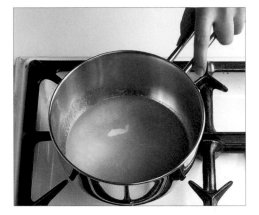

*2* Gently heat the half-fat spread in a saucepan, until melted.

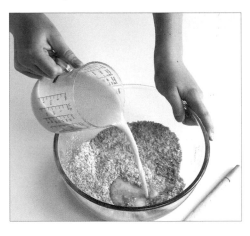

*3* Mix together the melted fat, sugar, egg and milk in a bowl, and pour over the dry ingredients.

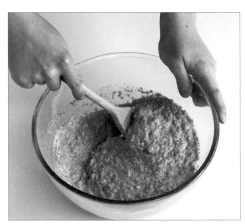

*4* Using a spoon or spatula, gently fold the ingredients together, but only enough to combine them. The mixture should look quite lumpy; overmixing will result in particularly heavy muffins.

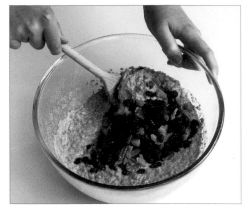

*5* Fold the pears and raisins into the mixture.

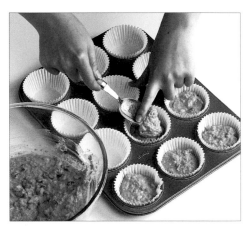

*6* Spoon the mixture in equal-sized portions into the prepared muffin or bun pans. Bake for approximately 15–20 minutes, until they are well risen and have turned golden brown. Turn the cakes out onto a wire rack and let cool before serving.

---

NUTRITION NOTES

Per portion:

| | |
|---|---|
| Energy | 108kcals |
| Protein | 3.40g |
| Fat | 2.68g |
| Saturated fat | 0.70g |
| Carbohydrate | 18.84g |
| Fiber | 2.64g |
| Added sugar | 4.37g |
| Sodium | 0.15g |

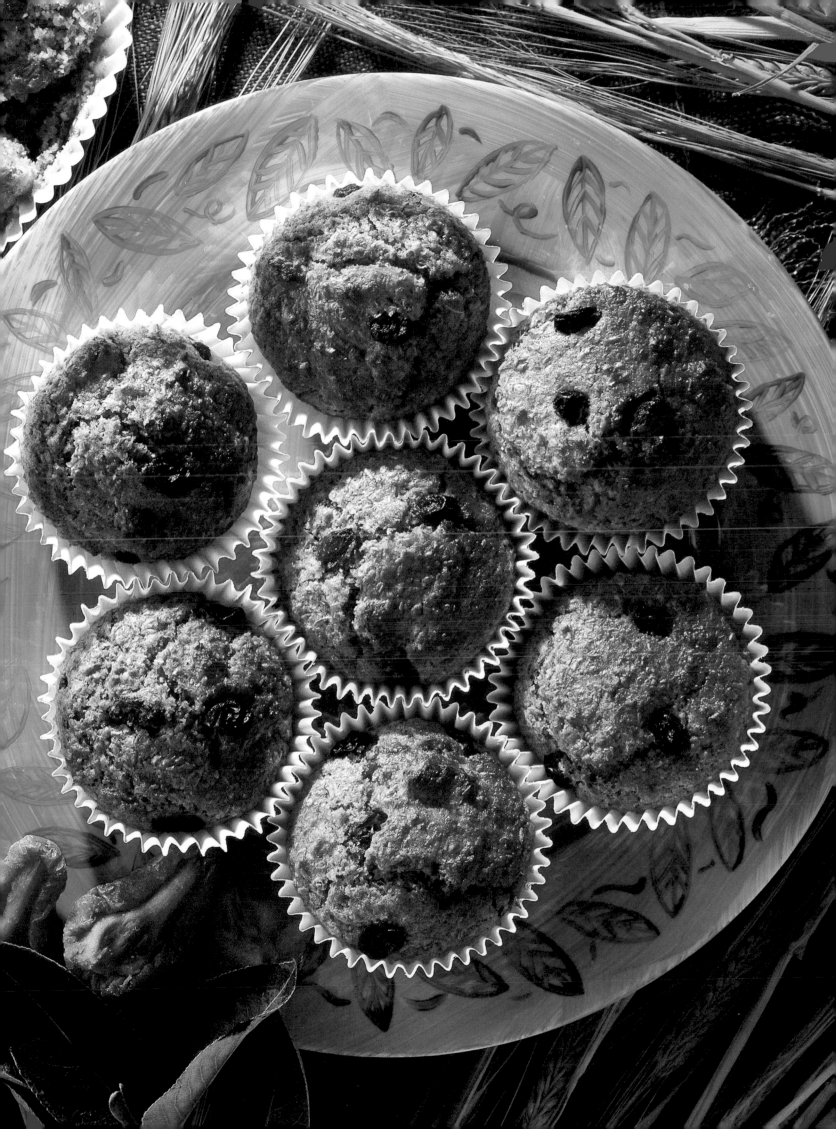

# Banana Bran Loaf

A tempting and filling teatime treat, this loaf is delicious served in slices, either on its own or with a little butter.

## INGREDIENTS

*Serves 12*
½ cup half-fat spread
½ cup light brown sugar
3 eggs, beaten
1½ cups whole-wheat flour, sifted
2½ cups bran
2 teaspoons baking powder, sifted
1 teaspoon salt
1–2 teaspoons ground ginger
3 medium bananas, mashed
1 cup raisins

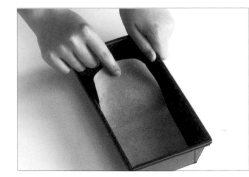

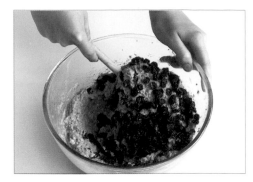

*1* Preheat the oven to 350°F. Lightly grease a 9 x 5 x 3-inch loaf pan, and line the bottom with baking parchment.

*2* Put the half-fat spread, sugar, eggs, flour, bran, baking powder, salt and ground ginger in a bowl, and beat together, using a wooden spoon or electric mixer, until it has been thoroughly mixed.

*3* Add the mashed bananas to the cake mixture and beat, until well mixed. Fold in the raisins.

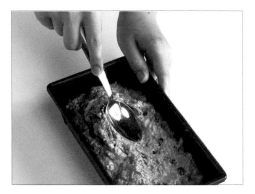

*4* Spoon the mixture into the prepared pan, and level the surface.

*5* Bake the loaf for about 1¼ hours, until it is well risen, golden brown and firm to the touch. Cool in the pan for a few minutes, then turn out onto a wire rack to cool completely. Serve in slices, either warm or cold, whichever you prefer.

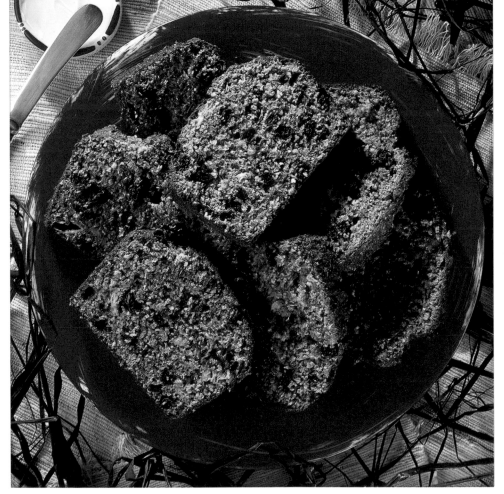

---

NUTRITION NOTES

Per portion:
| | |
|---|---|
| Energy | 211kcals |
| Protein | 5.42g |
| Fat | 6.11g |
| Saturated fat | 1.63g |
| Carbohydrate | 36.30g |
| Fiber | 3.40g |
| Added sugar | 9.71g |
| Sodium | 0.09g |

# Fruity Muesli Bars

These fruity muesli bars make an appetizing snack at any time of day. When they are cool, keep them moist by sealing them with plastic wrap.

## INGREDIENTS

*Makes 10–12*

8 tablespoons half-fat spread
⅓ cup light brown sugar
3 tablespoons golden or light
   corn syrup
1¼ cups Swiss-style muesli, with no
   added sugar
½ cup rolled oats
1 teaspoon pumpkin pie spice
⅓ cup golden raisins
½ cup dried pears, chopped

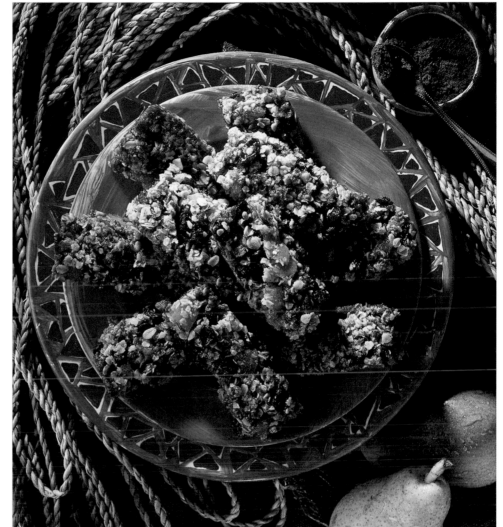

1 Preheat the oven to 350°F. Lightly grease a 7-inch square cake pan.

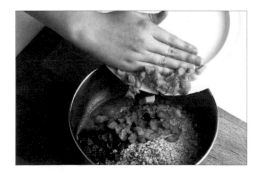

2 Put the half-fat spread, sugar and syrup in a saucepan, and gently heat until melted and blended, stirring.

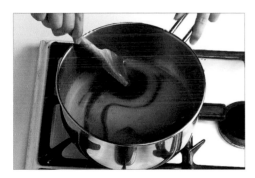

3 Remove the pan from heat, add the muesli, oats, spice, golden raisins and pears, and mix well.

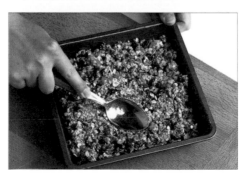

4 Transfer the mixture to the prepared pan and level the surface, pressing down.

5 Bake for 20–30 minutes, until golden brown. Cool slightly in the pan, then mark into bars using a sharp knife. When firm, remove the muesli bars from the pan and cool on a wire rack.

---

### NUTRITION NOTES

Per portion:

| | |
|---|---|
| Energy | 191kcals |
| Protein | 3.09g |
| Fat | 6.26g |
| Saturated fat | 1.59g |
| Carbohydrate | 32.57g |
| Fiber | 1.66g |
| Added sugar | 10.14g |
| Sodium | 0.11g |

---

### VARIATION

A combination of rolled oats and oatmeal can be used in place of muesli for a delicious change. The dried fruit helps to make the bars more naturally sweet.

# Carrot and Coconut Cake

A satisfying cake with a delicious combination of flavors.

## INGREDIENTS

*Serves 10*
½ cup half-fat spread
generous ½ cup superfine sugar
2 eggs
1½ cups whole-wheat flour, sifted
2½ cups bran
2 teaspoons baking powder, sifted
1 teaspoon salt
6 tablespoons skim milk, plus a little extra to mix
1⅔ cups carrots, coarsely grated
1 cup dried coconut
⅓ cup golden raisins
finely grated zest of 1 orange
1–2 tablespoons raw sugar

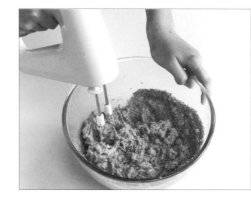

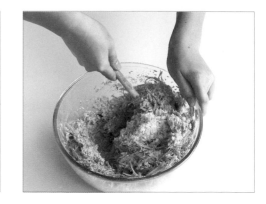

*1* Preheat the oven to 350°F. Lightly grease a deep 7-inch round cake pan and line with baking parchment. Put the half-fat spread, sugar, eggs, flour, bran, baking powder and milk in a large mixing bowl. Using an electric mixer, if you like, beat all the ingredients together, until they are thoroughly mixed.

*2* Fold in the carrots, coconut, golden raisins and orange zest, plus extra milk if needed, to make a soft dropping consistency.

*3* Spoon the mixture into the prepared pan, and level the surface.

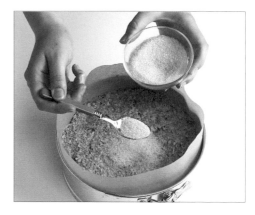

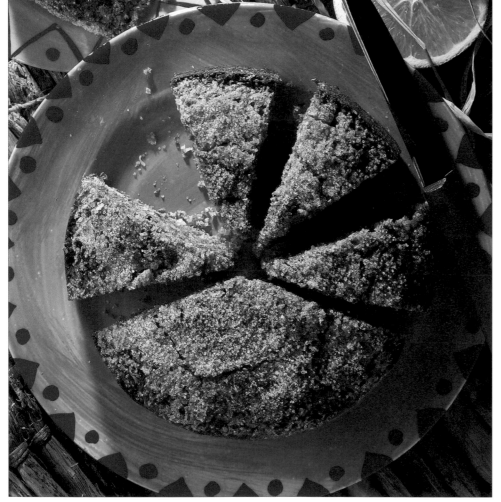

*4* Sprinkle the top with the raw sugar and bake for about 1 hour, until risen, golden brown and firm to the touch. Cool in the pan for a few minutes, then turn out onto a wire rack to cool completely before cutting it into slices.

| NUTRITION NOTES | |
| --- | --- |
| Per portion: | |
| Energy | 280kcals |
| Protein | 6.25g |
| Fat | 13.78g |
| Saturated fat | 7.91g |
| Carbohydrate | 35.17g |
| Fiber | 5.61g |
| Added sugar | 16.13g |
| Sodium | 0.11g |

# Farmhouse Apple and Golden Raisin Cake

A slice of this moist and lightly spiced fruit cake makes the perfect treat with a cup of tea. You could also have some for breakfast with plain yogurt.

## INGREDIENTS

*Serves 12*

¾ cup half-fat spread
¾ cup light brown sugar
3 eggs
2 cups whole-wheat flour, sifted
1 cup self-rising all-purpose flour, sifted
2 teaspoons baking powder, sifted
1 teaspoon salt
2 teaspoons pumpkin pie spice
12 ounces cooking apples, peeled, cored and diced
1 cup golden raisins
5 tablespoons skim milk
2 tablespoons light brown sugar

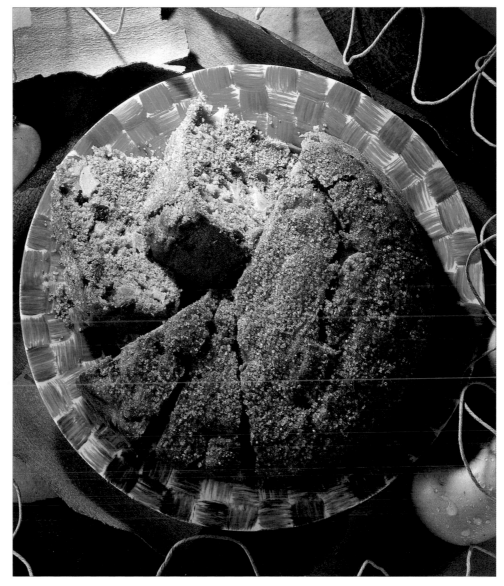

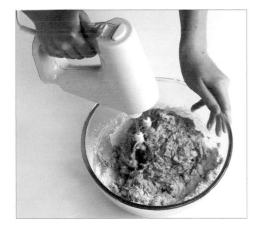

1 Preheat the oven to 325°F. Lightly grease a deep 8-inch round, loose-bottomed cake pan and line with baking parchment. Put the half-fat spread, soft brown sugar, eggs, flours, baking powder and spice in a bowl, and beat well together, until thoroughly mixed.

2 Fold in the apples, golden raisins and sufficient milk to make a soft dropping consistency.

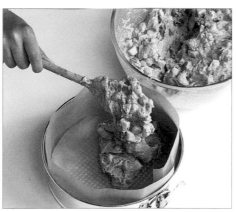

3 Spoon the mixture into the prepared pan, and make sure that the the surface is level and smooth. Sprinkle the top of the cake with a little brown sugar.

4 Bake for about 1½ hours, until risen, golden brown and firm to the touch. Cool in the pan for a few minutes, then turn out onto a wire rack to cool completely. Serve in slices.

| NUTRITION NOTES | |
|---|---|
| Per portion: | |
| Energy | 278kcals |
| Protein | 6.56g |
| Fat | 8.08g |
| Saturated fat | 2.16g |
| Carbohydrate | 48.55g |
| Fiber | 2.60g |
| Added sugar | 16.95g |
| Sodium | 0.16g |

# Cheese and Pineapple Whole-wheat Scones

These cheese and pineapple scones are delicious eaten freshly baked, either warm or cold, as you prefer.

## INGREDIENTS

*Makes 14–16*

2 cups self-rising whole-wheat flour, sifted
3 teaspoons baking powder, sifted
1 teaspoon salt
3 tablespoons polyunsaturated margarine
1 teaspoon mustard powder
¾ cup reduced-fat aged cheddar cheese, finely grated
¼ cup dried pineapple, finely chopped
⅔ cup skim milk

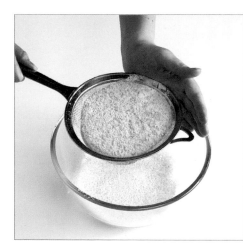

*1* Preheat the oven to 425°F. Line a baking sheet with baking parchment. Sift the flour, baking powder and salt into a bowl.

---

COOK'S TIP

---

For economy, grate the cheese finely so it will go further and you will use less.

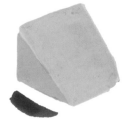

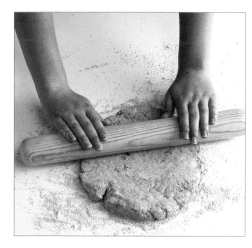

*2* Rub in the fat, until the mixture resembles bread crumbs.

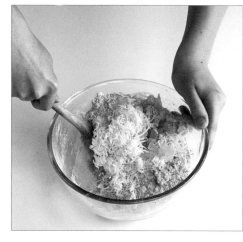

*3* Fold in the mustard powder, cheese and pineapple and stir. Add milk as needed to make a fairly soft dough.

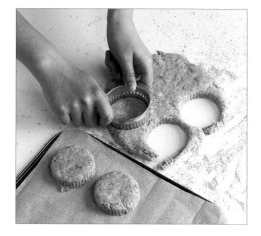

*4* Turn the dough onto a lightly floured surface and knead gently. Roll out to a thickness of ¾ inch.

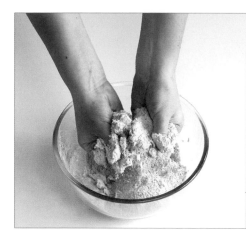

*5* Using a 2-inch fluted cutter, stamp out rounds and place them on the prepared baking sheet.

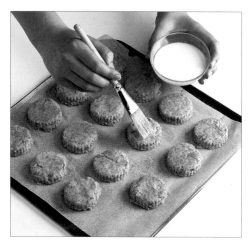

*6* Brush the tops of the scones with a little milk, and bake them for about 10 minutes, until they are well risen and golden brown. Transfer the scones to a wire rack to cool, and serve either warm or cold.

---

NUTRITION NOTES

---

Per portion:

| | |
|---|---|
| Energy | 99kcals |
| Protein | 4.22g |
| Fat | 3.62g |
| Saturated fat | 1.05g |
| Carbohydrate | 13.28g |
| Fiber | 1.74g |
| Added sugar | 1.33g |
| Sodium | 0.06g |

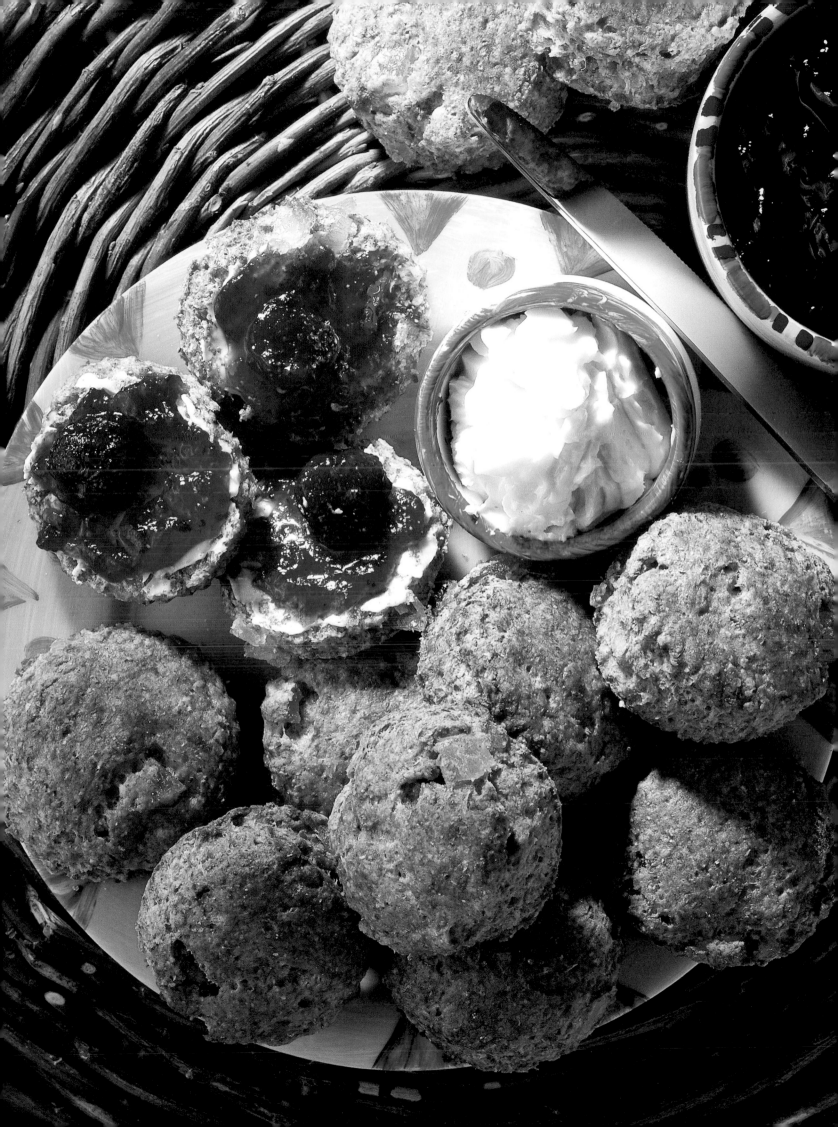

# Date and Orange Slice Bars

These tempting, wholesome slices are moist and chewy.

## INGREDIENTS

*Makes 16*

2 cups pitted dried dates, finely chopped
scant 1 cup freshly squeezed orange juice
finely grated zest of 1 orange
1 cup whole-wheat flour
1¾ cups rolled oats
½ cup fine oatmeal
pinch of salt
¾ cup half-fat spread
⅓ cup light brown sugar
2 teaspoons ground cinnamon

*1* Preheat the oven to 375°F. Put the dates in a saucepan with the orange juice. Cover, bring to a boil and simmer for 5 minutes, stirring occasionally.

---
VARIATION
---

Dried apricots or prunes used in place of the dates in this recipe make equally delicious slices.

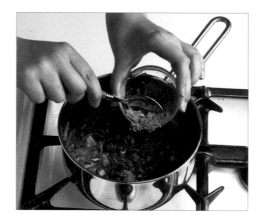

*2* Stir in the orange zest, and set aside to cool completely.

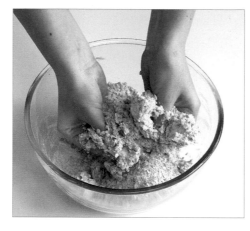

*3* Lightly grease a 7 x 11-inch nonstick baking pan. Put the flour, oats, oatmeal and salt in a bowl, and mix together. Lightly rub in the half-fat spread.

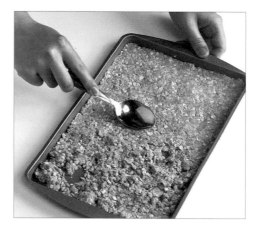

*4* Stir in the sugar and cinnamon. Place half the oat mixture on the bottom of the prepared pan and, using the back of a spoon, press it down firmly.

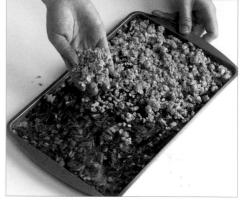

*5* Spread the date mixture on top and sprinkle the remaining oat mixture evenly over the dates to cover them completely. Press down lightly. Bake for about 30 minutes, until golden brown.

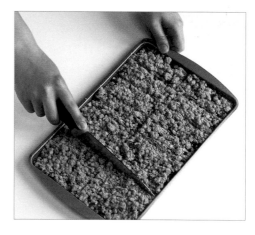

*6* Allow to cool slightly in the pan and mark into 16 pieces, using a sharp knife. When firm, remove the slices from the pan and cool completely on a wire rack. Finally, break the cooked fruit and oatmeal bars into fingers.

---
NUTRITION NOTES
---

Per portion:

| | |
|---|---|
| Energy | 197kcals |
| Protein | 4.02g |
| Fat | 5.76g |
| Saturated fat | 1.48g |
| Carbohydrate | 34.06g |
| Fiber | 1.76g |
| Added sugar | 5.25g |
| Sodium | 0.08g |

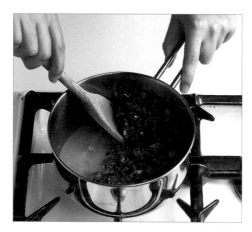

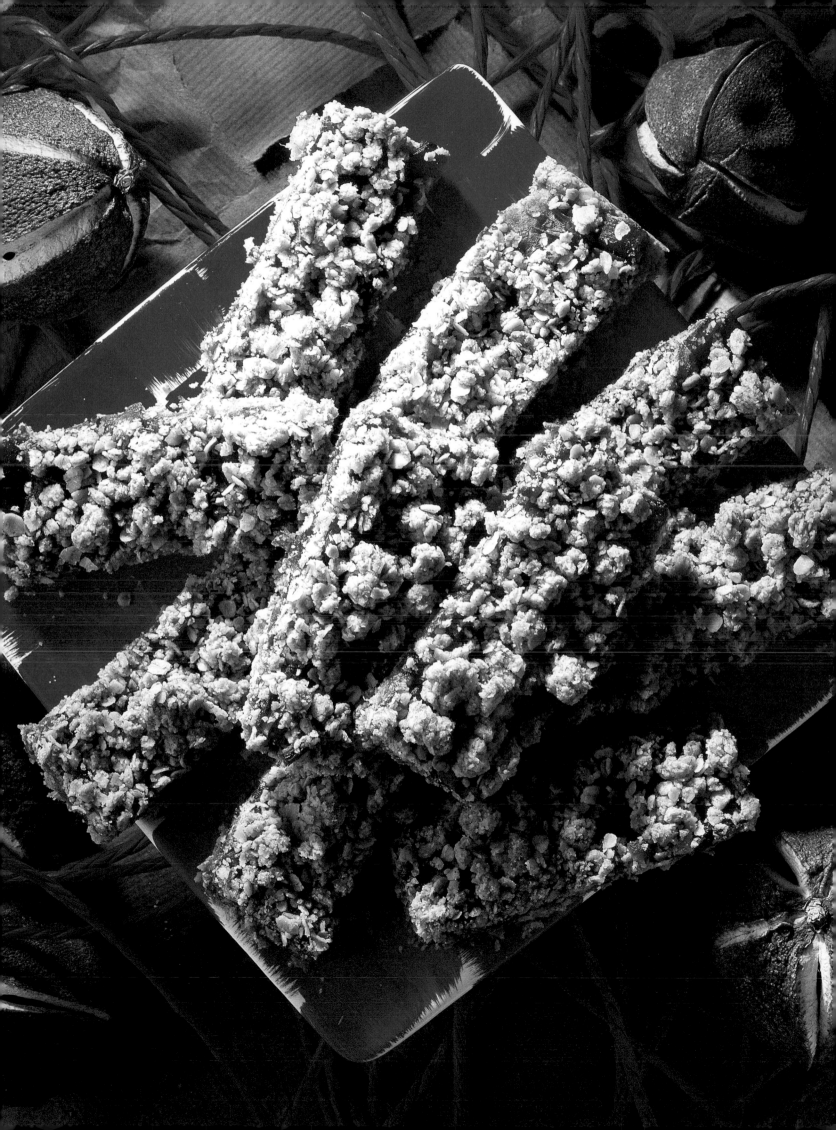

# Lemon and Raisin Rock Cakes

These lightly spiced, fruity rock buns (a British specialty) are easy to make, and delicious to eat.

## INGREDIENTS

*Makes 16*
2 cups whole-wheat flour
2 teaspoons baking powder
1 teaspoon salt
½ cup half-fat spread
generous ½ cup raw sugar
1 teaspoon pumpkin pie spice
finely grated zest of 1 lemon
⅔ cup raisins
1 egg, beaten
skim milk, to mix
pared lemon zest, to decorate

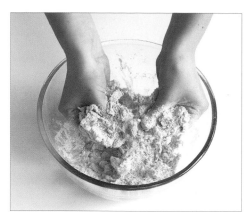

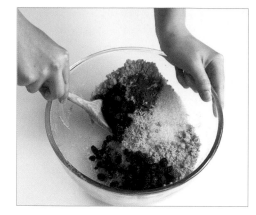

*1* Preheat the oven to 400°F. Line two baking sheets with baking parchment, and set aside. Put the flour and salt in a bowl, and lightly rub in the half-fat spread, until the mixture resembles bread crumbs.

*2* Add the sugar, spice, lemon zest and raisins to the flour mixture, and mix together.

*3* Stir in the egg and enough milk to make a stiff, crumbly mixture.

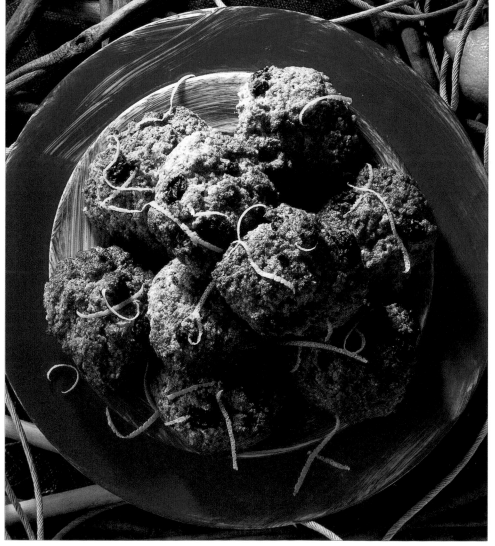

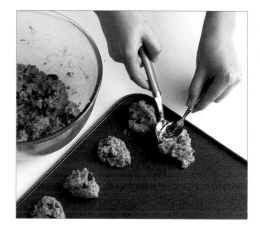

*4* Using two spoons, put rough heaps of the mixture onto the prepared baking sheets. Bake for 15–20 minutes, until lightly browned and firm to the touch. Transfer to a wire rack to cool. Serve decorated with lemon zest.

| — NUTRITION NOTES — | |
| --- | --- |
| Per portion: | |
| Energy | 126kcals |
| Protein | 2.90g |
| Fat | 3.64g |
| Saturated fat | 0.96g |
| Carbohydrate | 21.69g |
| Fiber | 1.41g |
| Added sugar | 7.55g |
| Sodium | 0.06g |

# Prune and Nut Tea Bread

Prunes, hazelnuts and walnuts make a successful partnership in this satisfying tea bread, which is also highly nutritious.

## INGREDIENTS

*Serves 12*

1½ cups pitted dried
  prunes, chopped
¾ cup light brown sugar
1¼ cups cold brewed tea
1 egg, beaten
½ cup hazelnuts, chopped
½ cup walnuts, chopped
2 cups whole-wheat flour
2 teaspoons baking powder
1 teaspoon salt
2½ cups bran

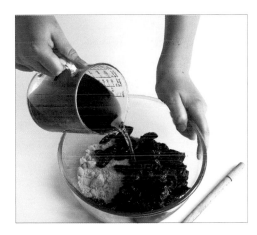

*1* Put the prunes, sugar and tea in a bowl, and mix together. Cover and let stand for about 4 hours, until most of the tea has been absorbed by the fruit.

| NUTRITION NOTES | |
|---|---|
| Per portion: | |
| Energy | 223kcals |
| Protein | 5.53g |
| Fat | 6.77g |
| Saturated fat | 0.67g |
| Carbohydrate | 38.17g |
| Fiber | 5.28g |
| Added sugar | 14.77g |
| Sodium | 0.02g |

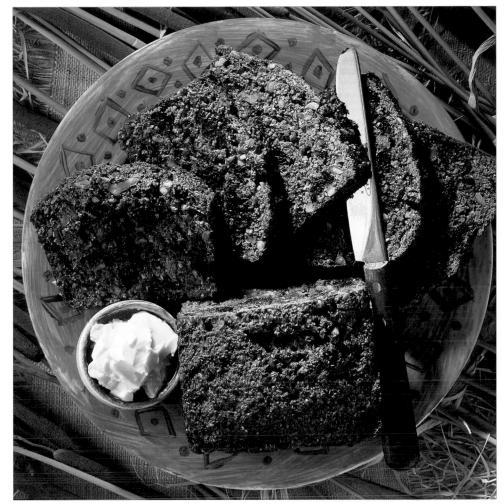

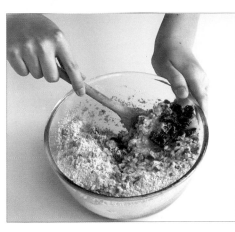

*2* Preheat the oven to 350°F. Lightly grease a 9 x 5 x 3-inch loaf pan. Add the egg, nuts, flour and bran to the prune mixture and, using a spoon, mix thoroughly.

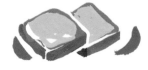

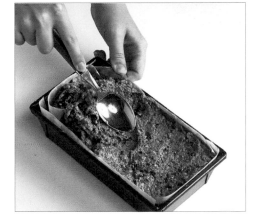

*3* Turn the mixture into the prepared pan, and level the surface.

*4* Bake for about 1¼ hours, then insert a skewer to check that the bread is cooked throughout. Cool in the pan for a few minutes, then turn out onto a wire rack to cool completely. Serve cut into slices.

# Cheese and Herb Whole-wheat Soda Bread

Full of flavor, this delicious, savory bread should be served freshly baked.

**INGREDIENTS**

*Serves 8*

3 cups whole-wheat flour
1 cup fine oatmeal
2 teaspoons baking soda
2 teaspoons cream of tartar
½ teaspoon salt
1 cup reduced-fat aged Cheddar
  cheese, finely grated
3–4 tablespoons chopped fresh
  mixed herbs
½ teaspoon mustard powder
1¼ cups buttermilk
water, to mix
2 tablespoons skim milk
1 tablespoon medium oatmeal

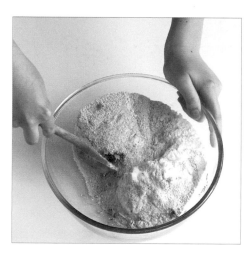

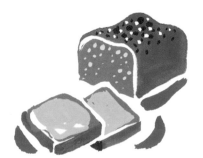

*1* Preheat the oven to 400°F. Lightly grease a baking sheet. Put the flour, oatmeal, baking soda, cream of tartar, salt, cheese, herbs and mustard powder into a bowl, and mix together.

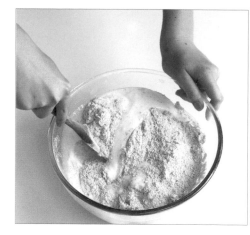

*2* Stir in the buttermilk and enough water to make a soft dough.

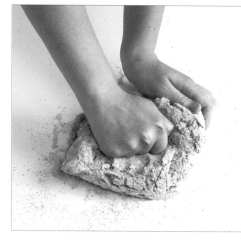

*3* Lightly knead on a floured surface. Shape into an 8-inch round.

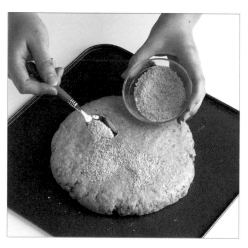

*4* Place the round of dough on the prepared baking sheet, brush the top with milk, and sprinkle evenly with medium oatmeal.

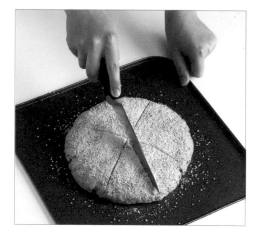

*5* Mark the top into eight even wedges. Bake for 30–40 minutes, until well-risen, firm to the touch and golden brown.

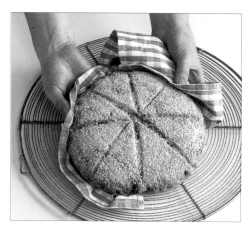

*6* Allow to cool on a wire rack. Break the soda bread into wedges to serve, and eat either warm or at room temperature, as you prefer.

| NUTRITION NOTES | |
| --- | --- |
| Per portion: | |
| Energy | 251kcals |
| Protein | 13.46g |
| Fat | 4.84g |
| Saturated fat | 1.87g |
| Carbohydrate | 40.94g |
| Fiber | 5.18g |
| Added sugar | 0.00g |
| Sodium | 0.25g |

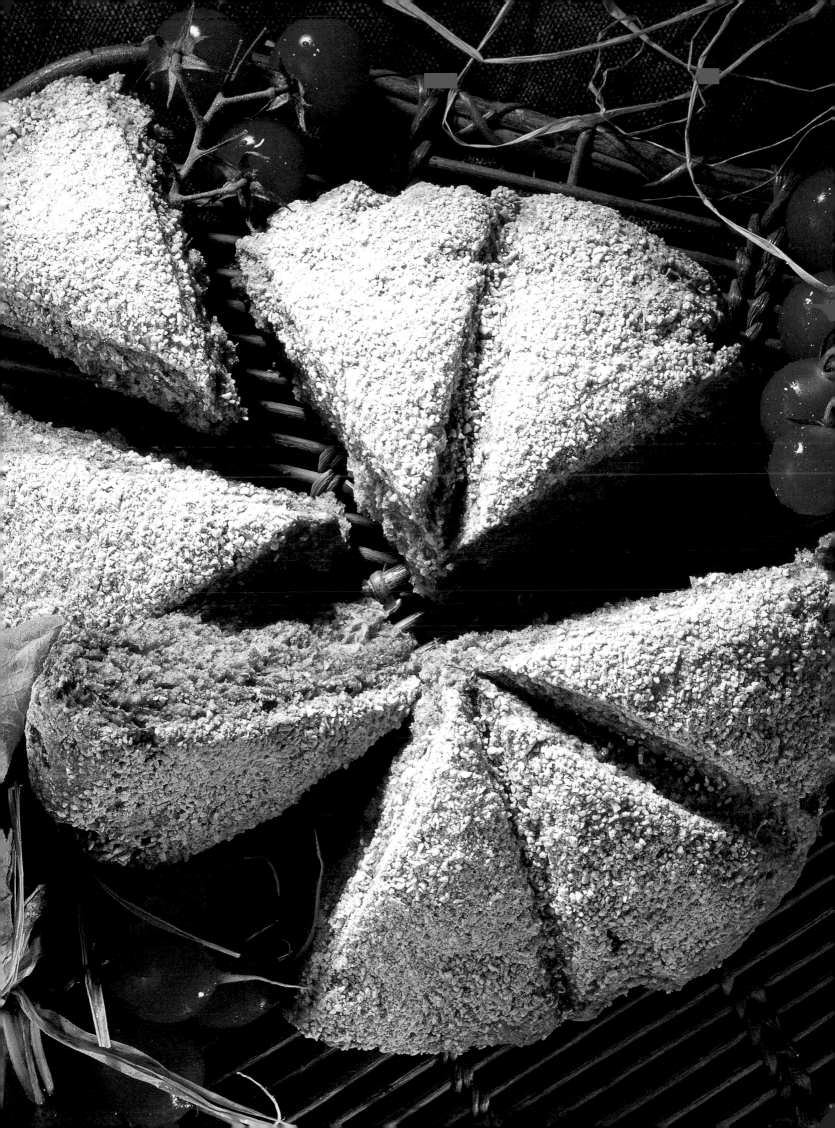

# INDEX